BEDLAM

....

BEDLAM

Greed, Profiteering, and Fraud in a Mental
Health System Gone Crazy

JOE SHARKEY

....

ST. MARTIN'S PRESS
NEW YORK

Design by Diane Stevenson / SNAP·HAUS GRAPHICS

Library of Congress Cataloging-in-Publication Data

Sharkey, Joe.
    Bedlam / Joseph Sharkey.
        p.   cm.
    "A Thomas Dunne Book."
    ISBN 0-312-10421-9
    1. Psychiatric hospitals—United States—Corrupt practices.
2. Hospitals, Proprietary—United States—Corrupt practices.
3. Mental health services—United States—Marketing—Corrupt
practices.   4. Psychiatric referral—United States—Corrupt
practices. I. Title.
RC443.S52   1994
362.2'1'0973—dc20   93-43386
                                                              CIP

A Thomas Dunne Book

First edition: April 1994

10 9 8 7 6 5 4 3 2 1

For Lisa

ACKNOWLEDGMENTS

....

I am indebted to a number of people whose names are not mentioned in the narrative of this book, especially the late Dr. Judson K. Albaugh, a brilliant and honorable psychiatrist who worked the tough end of the business, and who died while this was in progress. He was my father-in-law and my friend.

Thanks for research help are due to Mickey Uelses and Tim Morrison, staff investigators with the U.S. House of Representatives Select Committee on Children, Youth, and Families; Leslie Lemon, of the Texas Senate Committee on Health and Human Services; Ken Nichols, of the Texas Board of Private Investigators; Alison Tattersall; Mary Jane White; Jenny Labalme; Robert Thomas; Walt Malone, and Alison Duncan.

During 1991, certain reporters in Texas were especially tenacious in covering the scandals that came to light there. Prominent among them, I thought, were Bill Hendricks of the San Antonio *Express-News* and Mark Smith of the *Houston Chronicle*, who both sank their teeth into the story and didn't let go.

Two good and wise friends, Fred Brock and Joseph Beagan, provided crucial reality checks on important occasions during this endeavor. Thanks to my agent, Jane Dystel; my editor, Tom Dunne; to Christopher for being there; and, as always, to Nancy.

BEDLAM

....

INTRODUCTION

....

A DIFFICULT PERSONAL EXPERIENCE INDIRECTLY LED ME TO write this book. If it weren't for this relatively trivial encounter, I would probably remain unaware of how the for-profit psychiatric hospital industry and its collaborators in the profession of psychiatry have hijacked a multibillion-dollar segment of the American health-care market.

In the summer of 1990, with a twenty-year career as a news-paperman behind me and a couple of books under my belt, I finally faced a situation that I had been denying since my roistering days in college: I drank too much.

Now, I wasn't the sort of stumblebum, wild-eyed drunk like Ray Milland in *The Lost Weekend,* lurching down Third Avenue des-perate to pawn his typewriter. Few high-end boozers in the com-fortable early glow of middle age have hit that stage; some, in fact, never will. Smugly, some heavy drinkers can surround themselves with the loving family, toasting the good life from the leafy harbor of the backyard deck. Time is an ally, but time ran out for me that summer. My wife, Nancy, a woman whose capacity for love is fortunately exceeded only by her wisdom, had taken a hard look down the road as she contemplated middle age herself, and decided she wasn't ready to go all the way to the cliff with someone who showed every indication that he would end up as an elderly drunk. I had an odd flashback to a family Memorial Day party a few weeks earlier. It was a fleeting image, barely registered at the time, of my son, a happy and trusting boy of eleven ensconced in that ephemeral phase of preadolescence during which a kid still thinks his old man can outhit Babe Ruth. I saw him hoisting a Hires root beer bottle to his lips with a snappy flourish that he could only have learned from watching Dad guzzle a beer. A news flash from hell had just come in.

Initially, I believed that all of this had occurred without warning, but of course that's the usual story. The warnings had been in fact persistent over the years; suddenly, in hindsight, the sullen looks, angry tears, and the sickening glimmer of police-car lights in the rearview mirror one night came sharply into focus.

I'm not sure how to define what an alcoholic actually is, although I think I know one when I see one. At any rate, I've always suspected that stupidity had more to do with alcoholism than biology did. Certainly, drinking had become a problem in my life. I had spent years earnestly battling to moderate and sometimes conceal drinking, with a degree of success—none of my friends, for example, would have described me as a drunk—but it seemed to be shaping up as a losing fight. I had *liked* to drink; some of the most amusing times of my life were spent in the company of drink. But finally drinking had gone on long enough; value was no longer being delivered for the price. With middle age came new priorities, not to mention that ultimatum. I was damned if I was going to lose my wife and subject my children to the grim prospects of *Life with Father II: The Old Boozer.*

Luckily, there was a known cure. I stopped drinking, cold. Through no personal virtue other than having the good fortune to have married well and to have reached the second half of my life with most of my brain cells evidently in order, it turned out to be, in fact, as simple as that. Fortunately for me, the same cold black

Celtic mists that had probably incubated my environmental, if not genetic, predisposition toward excessive drink had also instilled the surly single-mindedness that allowed me to club the beast to death, once it was sufficiently exposed as my mortal enemy. Secretly, I roared at the rout.

But with the Choruses of Addiction at full voice in the America of the Recovery Era, I perceived a need to moderate my hubris. To oppose dogma was worse than heresy; it was Denial, the act that proves the intention of sin. I decided to do what was expected of me in modern America. First, I went to a couple of Alcoholics Anonymous meetings. With the scent of imminent damnation adrift like incense in those church basements, I tentatively joined people who talked, prayed, and—above all—proclaimed their eternal vulnerability. Over coffee, earnest souls reacted with quiet alarm when I mentioned that I hadn't had any problem stopping drinking once I saw that there was no future in it. Gravely, I was admonished that it was typical for a drunk to go on the wagon and then fall off during the victory celebration. In such circumstances, one cannot simply stop drinking and blithely continue with life unimpeded, they said. Grim emotional toil lay ahead; testimony must be offered, forgiveness beseeched, powerlessness humbly conceded. There would be penance, and attendance everlasting in the resolute assembly of the tenuously saved.

To hell with that, I decided. Even though there is general consensus that nonprofit support programs like Alcoholics Anonymous have by far the best track record in helping people to overcome alcohol problems—far better, say, than those $30,000-a-month "cures" in rehab—dedicated twelve-stepping wasn't for me. I said thanks and went my own way.

Still, I was intrigued by the experience. Resolved to investigate my options fully, I began looking into those alcohol-recovery programs that have been so popular, and so heavily marketed, during the past decade. Sure enough, Fair Oaks Hospital, in Summit,

New Jersey, not thirty minutes from my home in the New York City suburbs, boasted one of the most highly regarded alcoholism treatment programs in the East.

Thanks to years of heavy advertising and testimonials from celebrities such as Betty Ford, I knew that these places offered not only the intensive inpatient rehab regimens that yanked drunks and other addicts into sobriety with all the finesse of marine boot camp, but also outpatient programs that reinforced sobriety in one or two nightly sessions a week. And as the advertising for these programs invariably notes, health insurance usually pays for it all.

I wasn't especially amenable to spending a lot of my time, or even much of my insurance company's money for that matter, on unnecessary treatment. Like most Americans, I was well aware that medical costs were spinning out of control—the figure reached $939 billion in 1993, according to the Commerce Department, and is accelerating at a rate that will lift it to well over a trillion dollars in 1994.

What I did not even begin to imagine was how much of that money is being diverted into profit-making psychiatric and addiction facilities such as Fair Oaks and thousands of others. As the 1990s began (I subsequently learned), psychiatric treatment was identified by insurers as the fastest-growing segment of U.S. health-care costs. For businesses, the cost for providing mental health benefits (including treatment for alcoholism and drug addiction, which are often billed along with a secondary diagnosis of a mental disorder) has become one of the most out-of-control components of medical spending. Estimates used by the mental health "industry" itself—and it has come to see itself as an industry—were that in 1991 total costs for mental health care and addiction treatment exceeded $125 billion. By 1990, according to federal statistics, 25 percent of spending on employee health insurance went into psychiatric and addiction-treatment benefits.

Moreover, about 85 percent of that money was being channeled into inpatient hospital treatment—much of that in investor-owned

4

institutions that had clear profit incentives not only to entice as many patients as they could, but also to keep them as long as possible. Neither were these hospitals inconvenienced by the complicated restrictions that hamstring the general hospital business, since psychiatric care is virtually exempt from federal diagnostic-procedure guidelines. Yet this spending is accounted for by a small number of people. Fewer than 10 percent of those whose health insurance covers psychiatric and addiction treatment ever actually use those benefits.

No other country splurges so extravagantly on its medical bills. By the end of the 1980s, the United States was spending $2,354 a year per citizen—more than double the average sum spent by the twenty-four major industrial nations belonging to the Organization for Economic Cooperation and Development. In 1992, one out of every seven dollars in the U.S. economy—14 percent of gross domestic product—was spent on health care; this was nearly twice the average among the twenty-four OECD nations. But the money wasn't ensuring us the world's best health care. According to a survey published in late 1991 by *Health Affairs*, only four of those countries—Turkey, Greece, Portugal, and Spain—had higher infant-mortality rates than the United States. Only six had a lower life expectancy for males; eight had a lower life expectancy for females. Furthermore, the United States has the fourth-lowest ratio of inpatient hospital beds per 1,000 population.

Yet despite our stunning outlays, a large number of Americans are not covered by any form of health insurance. In 1993, of the country's 216 million people under age 65, about 37 million were without coverage. These are Americans living in households not poor enough to qualify for Medicaid, the $127-billion insurance program jointly funded by the states and the federal government, or not old enough for Medicare, the federal health insurance program for the elderly, which paid out $110 billion in 1991. By 1995, according to the National Governors Association, Medicaid will account for 28 percent of state budgets. And the Medicare program is facing insolvency as the population ages.

I have always instinctively understood the economic tenet that there is no such thing as a free lunch. Still, I was determined to at least explore the options, given my liberal health insurance benefits. I was open to the possibility of treatment. What did I have to lose? Bristling with resolve, receptive even to a therapeutic homily or two, I phoned Fair Oaks Hospital for information.

"You'll have to come in personally," said the businesslike woman who answered the hospital's phone. She asked me a series of questions, all of which seemed to be about finances and health insurance, but declined to provide any specific information about the hospital's programs. "It's our policy not to discuss these matters on the telephone, since everyone's recovery needs are different. Also, your wife has to come in with you," she said.

My wife? This seemed to be a very complicated way to dispense information—but my AA friends kept insisting that "denial" is a clear symptom of continued addiction, as is the need to control every situation. In my chastened state, I made an appointment and asked my wife to come along.

Fair Oaks Hospital occupies a wooded setting that, like most of the rest of New Jersey, is located just off a major highway. We arrived for our appointment after work on a balmy summer night; as we strolled up a winding drive from the parking lot, with the smell of fresh-mown grass in the air, I thought I saw a cluster of fireflies twinkling in the gloom of a glen near the path. But the pinpoint lights actually came from the tips of cigarettes in the hands of a group of people, evidently a recovery-treatment group out on a break. I could just make out the faces in the deep shadows— some of them young, hard-lined, with an indignant look suggesting that their owners had been sentenced there by a court. There also were a few women. One of them, who looked to be in her thirties, stood alone, staring at the ground, her shoulders hunched up as if against a chill, though the night was hot. I made brief eye contact with a man who appeared to be about my age. In a suit and tie, he had apparently come directly from work. He looked mortified and frightened, miserable beyond redemption.

My wife and I hustled inside. After a short interval in a brightly lit but otherwise deserted waiting room that might have belonged in a cardiologist's suite, a receptionist wearing a nurse's uniform led us in to a small, well-appointed inner office. There we faced an intense, rounded man in a gray suit with a pinstriped polyester tie. He sat at a desk writing on a sheet of paper.

My first impression, which I tried to suppress, was that we had just bought a car and that this was the salesman in the office at the back of the showroom where they take you to complete the paperwork and listen to the pitch about option packages. Had we been in an automobile showroom, every consumer defense mechanism I had would have been locked in place.

"Sit down, please!" our host said, getting up to position a chair in front of the desk for my wife, and gesturing me into one at the side. He introduced himself but already knew our names. He referred to a form on the desk, ticking off details of our insurance coverage, while murmuring what sounded like approval. My back stiffened. I knew my wife sensed this with some familiar alarm, so I forced myself to relax and look cordial.

Our interviewer, it transpired, was himself a recovering alcoholic, a "certified alcohol-abuse counselor," who said with a wink that he knew "all the tricks," including any I myself might be planning to use to avoid confronting the realities.

"Well, I think I might be over the biggest part already," I said modestly. "I've already stopped drinking—weeks ago, as I told the woman on the phone. Actually, as I said on the phone, we're really here for information about your outpatient program. I'm not sure it's something I want to go into, but if you wouldn't mind explaining a little—"

"A Pink Cloud," our man said, shaking his head ruefully.

7

"A what?"

"A Pink Cloud, that's what we call it. Every hotshot drunk who
quits drinking and thinks he has it licked, that's called going under
a Pink Cloud." He leaned toward me, and for the first time I noticed
a pockmarked face and watery blue eyes. His tone became harsh.
"You stop drinking, and you think that's all there is to it." He
snapped his fingers. "No freaking problem, right? Excuse my
French. What you're in right now, my friend, is a Pink Cloud,
which is nothing more than a Dry Drunk." He sat back and fixed
me with a stare that said I should be ashamed of myself. "You have
got a problem, my friend, and you're denying it to me and to your
wife."

Pink Cloud? Dry Drunk? This was the rhetoric of cultism, not
rational discourse. Only my desire not to alarm my wife kept me
from walking out on this character.

The interview continued for another half hour, varying in tone
among degrees of cajoling, reassurance, and a hard-edged insistence, which I found utterly baffling, that I was somehow deluding
myself into thinking I was well through with my problem. By this
point in our lives, my wife and I had been together long enough
that we didn't need to look at one another to know that we had
passed the point of diminishing returns—and possibly had mis-
takenly wandered into a comedy joint called the Pink Cloud. Curious now as to where this exercise was headed, we answered his
"counselor's" questions, determined to maintain at least the appearance of rapport with our equally determined salesman.

Yes, my wife said, she herself drank. A couple of beers here and
there, occasionally some wine with dinner. Seldom more than two
glasses. Had she ever been drunk? Oh, a couple of times in college,
maybe a little tipsy from time to time afterward. Like almost everyone else, she added, defensively. He scribbled notes.

Me? Well, of course, I had drunk assiduously for years, until I
stopped. Oh yeah, sure, some marijuana back in college, and of
course in Vietnam, where most of General Westmoreland's troops

8

had easy access to the best pot in the world. Nothing since then; I'd always preferred booze, even though it actually seemed more dangerous, and you always felt worse the next morning. Yes, to many of the other questions on his long list. I wasn't trying to hide the fact that drink had become a major problem in my life. I believed I was being given a personality test, and looked forward to hearing the results.

Laboriously, our interviewer jotted away on his forms, which I noticed were printed surveys, with spaces to tabulate scores. In one of the blanks, I could barely make out, upside down, what appeared to be the words "Ackwl subs. abuse."

Finally, our interlocutor toted up the individual and joint scores and announced the results. Surprise! I had failed the test. My "profile" indicated that I should be committed immediately in the twenty-eight-day, full-time, inpatient rehabilitation program. Along with my alcohol dependence I had racked up points on a whole host of psychological disorders and maladies; my suspicion of authority was apparently especially alarming, indicating, perhaps, a post-traumatic stress disorder associated with Vietnam, although the only combat I had ever seen was in a Saigon bar. I already knew how much money I would have to pay the hospital to get me "stabilized," as he put it—about $30,000. Fortunately, this would be fully covered by our health insurance policy.

But that wasn't all. The whole damn family, it transpired, was "indicated" for outpatient treatment for the pathological effects of "co-dependency," the emotional malaise of the 1980s.

It was pretty clear we weren't buying, and I had to give our interviewer credit for persistence. He probed for signs of vulnerability, but this was a set of radial tires he wasn't about to sell. We said we were leaving. With those imploring, watery blue eyes, he asked us to sign a form "so my boss knows I did my job and explained everything to you." Unwisely, we complied, eager to get out. We drove home, chuckling, but also wondering how many people, more desperate, alone, and vulnerable than I had been, might have succumbed to these tactics. We agreed I was doing just fine without transferring $30,000 of our insurance company's money to Fair Oaks. We didn't return our interviewer's follow-up phone calls.

Three weeks later, I was flabbergasted to get a bill from Fair Oaks Hospital, for $385, "for evaluation and diagnosis." I was also livid. It was as if a real-estate agent had sent a bill for showing a house. I wouldn't have trusted the man who interviewed us to "diagnose" my lawn mower; besides, I had gone there for information, not treatment. But we decided to let it go, not being inclined to do battle with a hospital's billing department. I sent the bill to Prudential, which paid it without a murmur.

Well over a year later, in the fall of 1991, I picked up *The New York Times* and read a story that described a disturbing situation. In Texas, New Jersey, Florida, Alabama, and elsewhere, it said, investigators had begun looking into widespread financial and ethical abuses by the private psychiatric hospitals that had sprung up by the hundreds all across the country during the 1980s, a time when extraordinary amounts of insurance money became widely available for mental-health and substance-abuse treatment. These psychiatric hospitals were accused of having "systematically misdiagnosed, mistreated and abused patients to increase profits from insurance claims," said the story. The terms "kidnapping" and "bounty hunters" leaped out from the gray columns of type. The article was one of the first—and, as it turned out, one of the last—comprehensive national news accounts about the situation, which quickly faded from public attention everywhere but in Texas, where state officials hammered away at the scandal for many months.

Yet the story resonated with me because of my own comparatively trivial experience with the salesman at Fair Oaks, a hospital that was not mentioned in the *Times* story. In the months that followed, I began looking more closely into what I have now come to see as one of the ugliest medical scandals in American history.

It became clear that many of these for-profit psychiatric facilities, mostly owned by rapidly expanding national hospital chains that were among the darlings of Wall Street in the 1980s, had been rapaciously preying for years on apprehensive, frightened people who were distressed enough to seek mental-health, addiction, or crisis counseling. These hospitals devised vast promotional programs—aggressive advertising coupled with painstaking media manipulation and systematic kickbacks to counselors and others who might have access to troubled potential patients—to create a whole new product niche: treatment in psychiatric wards for people who had never before been regarded as candidates for inpatient psychiatric care. As it had been used in past years to exploit anxieties about halitosis or dandruff, high-powered advertising was used to sell psychiatric treatment for emotional worries and behavioral difficulties. For the first time, in a virtually unregulated, profit-driven hospital environment, the principles of modern "guerrilla marketing" were being applied to psychiatric treatment, and with spectacular results.

In 1984, after an initial spurt of construction in the early part of the decade, there were 220 for-profit psychiatric hospitals in the United States. Four years later, as insurance money flooded into recovery treatment and psychiatrists devised new therapies based on a strategy of greatly expanding diagnostic definitions of what constitutes mental disorder—a process that resembled nothing so much as bid-rigging—the number of private psychiatric hospitals had more than doubled, to 444, according to the National Association of Private Psychiatric Hospitals. General hospitals, pinched by federal regulations limiting patient stays for medical procedures, also rushed to add psychiatric beds and to hire psychiatrists to come up with innovative programs to fill them. Joining in the expanding mental-health industry were literally thousands of profit-making psychiatric programs in general and community hospitals.

A 1990 national survey found that 40 percent of all U.S. hospital beds were occupied by psychiatric and substance-abuse patients. By 1990, the U.S. was spending far more on inpatient psychiatric care than on treating cancer.

To the booming psychiatric industry, some regions of the country, such as the Sunbelt, were particularly attractive, especially when state officials could be persuaded to relax restrictions on hospital construction. States such as Texas, Arizona, Nevada, Florida, and California were psychiatric gold mines in the 1980s. In Texas, for example, a robust economy coupled with a large population of military dependents yielded a vast pool of well-insured potential patients—and the number of private psychiatric hospitals tripled, reaching ninety, during the 1980s. Such hospitals depend almost exclusively on patients who have corporate or military health insurance. On the other hand, Texas finished the decade ranking forty-eighth among the fifty states in public spending on mental illness and substance abuse.

All over the country, kids are especially attractive customers— if their parents have insurance and can be enticed to commit them to a mental hospital. Between 1980 and 1987, the number of youths aged ten to nineteen who spent time confined to psychiatric hospitals soared 43 percent, according to federal statistical analyses. In one state, Illinois, the number increased fivefold. Ira Schwartz, a University of Michigan professor who is one of the leading national authorities on youth policy, told me that he believes this aspect of the psychiatric-hospital business constitutes "the biggest child-welfare scandal of the last fifty years."

But adults also provided brisk business for the modern profiteers, whose zeal in exploiting emotional misery dwarfed that of the supervisors of St. Mary of Bethlehem, the notorious English asylum Bedlam, where in the 18th century spectators were charged an admission fee to see the lunatics. At least Bedlam provided free care. In modern America, as severely mentally ill people are abandoned to roam the streets, investor-owned psychiatric institutions operate "800-number" telephone hot lines that entice callers with offers of help for emotional or substance-abuse problems—and, once insurance coverage is verified, sometimes pressure them to commit themselves or a relative to a mental institution. In recent years, competition for patients became so intense that U.S. corporate psychiatric hospitals opened recruitment offices in Canada to exploit loopholes in that country's national health insurance.

In Texas, the only state that has so far moved aggressively against psychiatric-hospital abuses, state senator Mike Moncrief said, "We discovered instances where social workers, school counselors, probation officers, crisis hot line workers, and even ministers were paid to refer paying patients to private psychiatric hospitals—people in our communities we have all been taught to trust, not to avoid."

These scams existed with the cooperation of a significant segment of American psychiatry, a profession that has always had to scramble for remuneration and professional respect. Thousands of psychiatrists forged financial links with psychiatric hospitals during the 1980s, often with the stated understanding that "diagnoses" were expected first to serve the need of the hospital to keep the "patient census" up. The potential for profit was staggering—some hospitals' staff psychiatrists were earning a million dollars a year and more, thanks to fees for signing diagnoses and to bonuses based on filling the beds.

Some critics insist that the modern psychiatric profession itself, and not just a few bad apples, is to blame. "Psychiatrists created this mess themselves by subscribing to and going along with the nefarious schemes of these hospital corporations," said Dr. Duard Bok, a psychiatrist who was fired by a psychiatric hospital after objecting to what he considered treatment abuses. "If we hadn't compromised our ethics, this never would have happened." Dr. Walter E. Afield, a psychiatrist who taught at Harvard and Johns Hopkins and founded a Florida company that reviews psychiatric treatment, said: "Enormous costs are being incurred and enormous profits are being generated. The abuse boggles the mind."

13

Psychiatric profiteering is driven by lavish liberalization of insurance coverage made available by the imperatives of the Recovery Era, in an atmosphere where burgeoning television talk shows and newspaper "lifestyle" sections accept without skepticism virtually any claim having to do with the notion that we are a nation of dysfunctional people in need of outside intervention in order to become mentally healthy. And so recovery gurus such as John Bradshaw have been able to redefine all of modern America as a pathological society in which "approximately 96 percent of the families are dysfunctional to one degree or another."

At the same time, those who stood to profit from this media-induced social narcissism worked insidiously to control the agenda in the places where the money was channeled. In 1970, health insurers were required by state or federal laws to cover thirty benefits; today, such benefits number over eight hundred—and various mandated psychiatric and substance-abuse benefits account for over half of them. Furthermore, it is now a firmly established principle of federal mental-health *policy* that in any six-month period, at least 20 percent of Americans are suffering from a diagnosable mental illness. The federal government has designated the 1990s the "Decade of the Brain," and funneled most mental-health research funding toward the interests of a biologically oriented psychiatric establishment working overtime to establish mental disorders and emotional disruptions as physical diseases that can be "cured" only with drugs and expensive medical intervention.

The historical ironies in the health-care crisis are compelling. Tuberculosis is back, with what *The New York Times* called in 1992 "strains so virulent they threaten to return pockets of American society to a time when antibiotics were unknown." The resurgence comes after two decades of sharp budget cuts in public-health programs. "Without these cuts, experts say, the disease could have been all but eradicated," *The Times* reported. Americans spent $67 billion on prescription drugs in 1990, but in providing polio vaccinations for one-year-olds, the United States now ranks seventeenth in the world—behind Albania, China, Mexico, and Pakistan.

Meanwhile, as we divert vast amounts of health-care money into mental-health treatment for those who have insurance, many of the genuinely mentally ill are not receiving adequate treatment and can now be found more readily in the streets and in jails than in hospitals. Moreover, as Americans face the prospect of sharp curtailments in health-care services, corporate psychiatry is gearing up, with encouragement from the well-established federal policies that define all mental illnesses as biological in nature, to sharply increase its influence over the routine administration of medical treatment in hospitals and even physician's offices.

A 1992 lawsuit by a group of major insurance companies against one leading chain of psychiatric hospitals called what has been going on in the mental-health industry "one of the most massive and pernicious health care scandals of all time."

I kept thinking of that $385 my insurance company paid to a hospital where I had gone just for information. The haunting image of a man and a woman dragging furtively on cigarettes in the summer gloaming also stayed in my mind. Obviously, what I had experienced was a tiny piece of the tale, hardly significant in the whole range of cynical manipulation of vulnerable people. But the audacity and cool efficiency of the hustle stuck with me. For example, I was amazed at how quickly my name had obviously been sold to outside mailing lists. Suddenly, my mailbox was full of solicitations about treatments for the whole range of maladies commonly associated with alcoholism, from heart disease and kidney trouble to depression, bad credit, and finally death. After some months, my wife started getting solicitations from mausoleums and estate planners, suggesting that she prepare herself for the inevitable.

Reporters tend to focus best when they are moved to indignation by injustice, hypocrisy, or chicanery. The more I thought about my experience, which was really an annoying combination of all three, the more determined I became to find out what was going on and (this thanks to a number of cynical years spent in financial journalism) exactly who was making a buck on it. Two books got my immediate attention. One, *The Diseasing of America: Addiction Treatment Out of Control,* by a clinical psychologist named Stanton Peele, impressed me with its blunt assessment of the overblown claims and pseudoscientific trappings of what Peele dismisses as "old and familiar moralism, albeit dressed in contemporary medical garb." The other, *Toxic Psychiatry,* by a psychiatrist named Peter R. Breggin, helped me to understand that expensive inpatient addiction-treatment scams were only one aspect of a medical scandal that involves the entire profession of psychiatry, which has allied itself with the drug and hospital industry and coopted the federal mental-health establishment in an unholy alliance to ensure profits by vastly expanding the definition of what constitutes mental illness—and how much health-insurance money should be poured into it.

Writing in *The Atlantic* in 1992, Arnold S. Relman, M.D., the former editor of the *New England Journal of Medicine,* warned of a growing "medical-industrial complex" producing a glut of hospital facilities and physicians. "With insurance available to pay the bills," he said, "physicians have powerful economic incentives to recruit patients and provide expensive services." I came to believe that this was especially true in the area of mental health. With few clear definitions of what is considered mental illness, marketing is being utilized not only to sell, refine, and expand established areas of treatment, but to invent whole new areas of "functional impairment" that will qualify for insurance reimbursement.

As America struggles to come up with genuine health-care reform—an undertaking that the Clinton administration policymakers have correctly called the biggest federal social-policy initiative since Social Security—the biopsychiatric-industrial complex is busily rewriting the definitions of mental illnesses. These definitions are in the hands of the people who have the most to gain from the claim (now accepted as doctrine by the psychiatric establishment) that familial, social, political, and educational crises are often rooted in physical imbalances in the brain. The psychiatric industry is working hard to expand and mandate insurance coverage to pay for biopsychiatry's new frontier. In 1990, for example, California became the first state to define mental illnesses as medical diseases and require that any health-insurance policy covering physical diseases of the brain also offer the same level of coverage for "schizophrenia, schizo-affective disorders, bipolar and delusional depressions and development disorder."

Born in a narcissistic era, nurtured by advertising, marketing, and media hype that promote even the most specious assertions about addiction, depression, and anxiety, the biopsychiatric-industrial complex is on the march. It prospers, like the fabled military-industrial complex, in direct proportion to the perceived threat. Consider the claim, currently respectfully received in biopsychiatric circles, that a third of the human population might be suffering from a single worldwide depressive disorder that is biochemical in origin—and, of course, curable with medicine. It's enough to make you miss the worldwide communist menace.

In the spring of 1992, during congressional hearings on profiteering by the psychiatric-hospital business, U.S. Representative Patricia Schroeder quoted from a Justice Department briefing: "Current intelligence shows that psychiatric hospitals and clinics are defrauding government programs and private insurers of hundreds of millions of dollars annually."

I now realize that the field of mental health, like human psychology itself, is riddled with hidden agendas. As I traveled around the country researching this book, I expected my journey to be cynical and arduous, and in many ways it was. But I was also left with an abiding impression of the people who came forward—not only former patients, but career hospital professionals, politicians, community workers, and even psychiatrists—to take a stand and say that what they had witnessed was an abuse of power, and that it was *wrong*. Their names will be found throughout this book. They are citizens who refused to countenance an intolerable situation, even when they were alone, with nothing to gain and plenty to lose. To me, that is a pretty good definition of courage. Meeting them renewed my faith in the common decency, and common sense, of America.

CHAPTER ONE

....

"SECTOR ONE" WAS JUST A NAME THAT JOHN WAYNE BLANKS
came up with in 1987 when he started his company.

It sounded like a terrific title for a television police series: "Sector
One," much more dramatic than "Rent-a-Cop"—which was, however, a more accurate description of John Wayne Blanks's new
business. At first, until it got involved in the hauling of people to
the psycho ward for between $150 and $450 per delivery, Sector
One's main activity was supplying security guards and night watch-
men to small companies, banks, and job sites in booming San
Antonio, Texas, during the later years of that Sunbelt metropolis's
remarkable decade-long growth spurt in the eighties.

Sector One started out well enough, but it soon became clear
to Blanks, who was quick to spot opportunities, that there was
plenty of room for much more significant growth. Blanks knew that
the key to entrepreneurial success was the ability to identify and
capture the new markets that were opening up all over the Southwest, in formerly sleepy little places that had been the greatest
beneficiaries of both the policies of the Reagan era and the population migration to the South and Southwest.

Blanks's opening was in the local and county offices, where he
realized that budget cuts were doing more than all the reform drives

in political history to shake the foundations of these once mighty fortresses of job patronage. The buzzword was "privatization"; for the first time in anybody's memory, politicians were actually forced to lay off workers and look to do things more cheaply in the private sector. Hiring part-time cops looking for moonlighting work, as well as ex-servicemen looking for any job they could get, Blanks began piling up contacts to put his security guards in the offices of government agencies and nonprofit groups in Bexar County, of which San Antonio is the seat.

Some of the best jobs were at homeless shelters, where Sector One's guards helped to keep things under control. From there, it was a logical step into public mental-health centers—and again, for some of the same reasons, there were few complaints about overstepping of authority.

In October 1989, largely because his guards had become so familiar at county agencies, Blanks managed to get Sector One into the county Mental Health and Mental Retardation Department's Crisis Stabilization Center, a nonprofit facility that provided immediate care for a wide range of emergencies. The center's clientele ranged from people on bad drug trips and severe alcohol benders to women and children who came in battered by husbands and parents.

In the atmosphere of constant crisis that prevails at such a place, it is easy to allow the lines of authority to become somewhat blurred. As at every other public-health facility in America, the center's staff were reeling from chronic money troubles. "When the copy machine broke down, there was no money to fix it, so we were running down to the 7-Eleven to use the five-cent copier they got there," one exasperated nurse recalled. The financial problems at the center, which handled about twenty thousand cases a year, went far beyond the copy machine, of course. By 1990, there wasn't even enough in the budget to continue funding one of the most important programs the center had—providing ambulance and taxicab service to pick up the desperate people who called the hot line asking urgently for help.

As a private contractor already on site, Blanks pondered the dilemma. "Budget constraints and the absence of other reasonable options presented little hope that the situation would improve," he would say later. He decided to step in. He purchased at auction three used police cruisers and had them marked with the words "Sector One" and official-looking insignia on their doors. These he used to provide the center's emergency transportation needs. Since Blanks charged about half of what the former ambulance and taxi system had, the center was glad to have him on the job.

So now Sector One security guards were going out into the community on emergency calls. By way of medical training, Blanks explained, the officers were told about psychiatric "diagnostic criteria" and "familiarized and briefed insofar as symptoms to recognize in certain categories of mental illness."

Blanks, with a bureaucrat's love of campaigns and programs, called this service the "Mobile Crisis Response Program." Suddenly, Sector One rent-a-cops, several of whom he promoted to the newly created rank of "security lieutenant," were rushing around San Antonio with lights flashing and sirens wailing, responding to emergencies like a psychiatric SWAT team.

Since the authority of Sector One's security guards, once they left the premises they were hired to protect, was questionable, Blanks and county mental-health officials drew up special legal authorization, which they christened the "Application for Emergency Detention Program." In the budget-crisis atmosphere, they easily got this program approved by a court magistrate. Unilaterally, it conferred on Blanks's rent-a-cops sweeping emergency powers that exceeded in scope even the arrest powers of real, on-duty police officers. Under its provisions, a Sector One security guard was permitted to make out an application for the emergency detention of any person, if the guard decided that person was having a mental-health or a substance-abuse crisis, and to take that person into custody at an approved mental-health facility, even if that person did not want to go. Court approval of the detention was required only after a twenty-four-hour period (or, in the case of detentions occurring on Friday, after the weekend).

The full scope of the new powers wasn't immediately clear. "When we first started, it was just a straight transportation service," Blanks later explained. "We would merely go to the residence or another location of a person who had voluntarily requested to be transported to a hospital."

John Wayne Blanks was born in Berkeley, California, in 1951 and quickly found his vocation. Immediately after graduation from high school in 1969, he got a job with the Los Angeles school district as a narcotics agent who posed as a student to provide information on drug use. He later did the same work at a small college in Oregon, where he provided information to the local police.

After a few years working as a small-town police officer in Idaho, Blanks ended up in Texas, where he worked for a year as an oil-field roughneck before landing a job as an equipment operator and salesman. After the decline of the oil business, Blanks worked as a prison guard for a while, and then finally turned to private se-curity-guard work in the San Antonio area, where one former boss described his duties as involving chiefly administration, personnel, payroll, "billing and collections," and "marketing new business." In October 1987, he went out on his own with Sector One.

Opportunities beckoned. During the 1980s, as San Antonio's population jumped by more than 250,000 to its current level of about 1 million, private psychiatric hospitals went on a growth spree to take advantage of the region's robust economy and attractive demographics. Unemployment was low, meaning health-insurance coverage rates were high. There were lots of well-insured military dependents taking advantage of liberal mental-health benefits. In fact, the overall cost to the federal government for mental-health care for military dependents shot up 126 percent between 1985 and 1989, which happened to be the years of the biggest building boom in private psychiatric hospitals.

The region has a large population of young people, who are major customers of the substance-abuse and family-crisis programs that are staples of private psychiatric care. An amazing two thirds of the population of San Antonio was under thirty-five years old by the middle of the eighties—and what's more, out in the well-tended suburbs, even the retired folks tended to be fairly young. With at least a dozen military facilities and bases dotting the area, many of those people were military retirees embarked on their second careers—comfortable family people with generous government health insurance in place for life.

The psychiatric hospitals lunged. In San Antonio, the number of private psychiatric hospitals jumped from two to nine in the four years from 1986 to 1990.

Logically enough, given his new expertise and what he called his "growing reputation" at the county Crisis Stabilization Center, Blanks—who referred to himself as a "skilled mental health hostage negotiator" on applications—turned his attention to the private psychiatric hospitals. Correctly claiming that Sector One already provided the only formal mental-health mobile crisis-response program in Bexar County, he approached the psychiatric hospitals and made his pitch, careful to explain the authority that his officers now had to detain people involved in psychiatric emergencies.

By 1990, with the recession locking in, the private psychiatric-hospital chains were receptive to the message. The growth had started to slow as corporate insurance providers were trimming spending on arbitrary psychiatric treatment. Hospitals fiercely competed to keep beds filled and profits up, while working off the weighty debt loads that were the main legacy of the previous decade's building frenzy. At the same time, while money was pouring into the high end of the psychiatric and substance-abuse business, public mental-health clinics and psychiatric emergency rooms had been hobbled by budget cutbacks, leaving many seriously mentally ill people to fend for themselves. This had so overwhelmed law enforcement that some police agencies simply stopped responding to reports of disruptive mentally ill people.

In no time at all, with contracts from four for-profit psychiatric hospitals, a private enterprise like Sector One was a force to be reckoned with in the mental-health care of Bexar County. Though Sector One had thirty employees, many of them moonlighting cops, only three—none of them police officers—were involved in what Blanks liked to refer to "hostile situations"—that is, taking people against their will to psychiatric hospitals. Those three were Officers Joe F. Saenz, Ulysses Jones, and their boss, Blanks himself.

Out in Live Oak, Texas, a quiet suburb beside I-35 just beyond the city limits northeast of San Antonio, Marianne Harrell and her fourteen-year-old grandson Jeramy had never heard of Sector One until the afternoon of April 12, 1991, when one of its emergency cars pulled into the driveway of their home, a ranch house in a leafy subdivision with a U.S. and a Texas flag on the pole in the side yard. The Harrells had legal custody of their grandsons, Jeramy and his two brothers.

Like many of their neighbors living in the well-kept ranch houses along the winding streets of Live Oak, the Harrells were retired military. Their grandsons' names were Rick, eighteen; Jeramy, fourteen; and Jason, twelve years old, and the only one who gave the Harrells significant grief.

Sid Harrell had spent twenty-three years as a medical technician in the Army, retiring with the rank of staff sergeant. As everybody always said, you could retire from the service after you did your twenty or thirty years, but you couldn't really leave it. Like many other retired military families, the Harrells never broke out of the gravitational field of the military installation. In their case, it was Fort Sam Houston, the sprawling base a half hour's drive into the city along the Pan-Am Expressway. Retirees like the Harrells routinely drove down to Fort Sam to shop in the commissary and post exchange, gas up the car, and, when necessary, take advantage of the free medical care at Brooke Army Medical Center, one of the best military hospitals in the country.

But even military hospitals had begun to cut back, and that was one of the reasons why Jason, the rambunctious one, happened to be undergoing treatment in a private psychiatric hospital on the afternoon the Sector One car pulled up.

Jason's main problem, as his parents saw it, was that he kept cutting school and running away from home. He wouldn't go far. He'd usually turn up downtown, where they'd find him hanging out someplace like Brackenridge Park, not far from the Alamo. There he'd be, defiant but hungry, planted on a bench under a moss-covered oak tree, watching the ducks in the pond.

The most recent time he played hooky, a police officer found him first, downtown as usual. When the officer inquired why he was not in school, the boy replied that his grandfather occasionally hit him. This got him taken directly to a Baptist home for runaways, where he faced an overworked child-abuse counselor. An hour or so after the boy was brought in, this counselor phoned the Harrells to say where Jason was and why. The boy was claiming that his grandfather was too strict.

The boy was obviously disruptive and troubled, the counselor said, the proof of which was that he had cut school and run away from home. He suggested that the Harrells consider sending the boy to a good private hospital, one with a program for troubled adolescents.

On the extension, the boy's mother quickly chimed in, "We can't afford a private hospital."

"Of course you can. You got the CHAMPUS, don't you?"

CHAMPUS is short for Civilian Health and Medical Program of the Uniformed Services. It's the federal health-insurance program that covers spouses and children of people in the military, and also retired military personnel and their families. In the realm of health insurance, CHAMPUS is Texas-sized: In the 1991 fiscal year, it paid out $631 million in psychiatric benefits. CHAMPUS's mental-health coverage, which included thirty days a year of in-patient care for adults and forty-five days for children, has been growing robustly. From 1980 to 1992, the number of people using CHAMPUS psychiatric benefits increased by 74 percent. Nationally, about 22 percent of CHAMPUS's $2.8 billion went toward mental-health treatment, mostly in private psychiatric facilities. However, Texas private mental hospitals were so well positioned that they managed to take in twice that average—or about *44 percent* of total CHAMPUS outlays in the state during 1990. San Antonio's private psychiatric hospitals received $1 out of every $20 CHAMPUS spent in Texas for psychiatric services.

"Yeah, we got the CHAMPUS," Marianne informed the Baptist Home counselor. It was just the kind of benefit a woman puts up with twenty years of raising a family in the Army to get, because you keep it till the day you die.

"Well, you're golden, then," the counselor declared. "You want me to give y'all a recommendation of a fine place to send the boy, your Jason? For his evaluation?"

"I reckon," Sid said uneasily.

"Well, you want to get him to Colonial Hills in San Antonio, the very best that there is. It's fully covered for CHAMPUS. I wouldn't recommend no place else, Mr. and Mrs. Harrell." Colonial Hills Hospital was owned by Psychiatric Institutes of America, the big national chain of mental hospitals. (PIA was in turn a subsidiary of a California hospital company called National Medical Enterprises Inc.)

All the Harrells knew then, however, was that the man at the Baptist Home had given them advice in a crisis, which they assumed to be good advice, and so it was settled. That afternoon, Sid Harrell drove over to the Baptist Home and picked up his very unhappy twelve-year-old. A little later, the grandparents took the boy down to Colonial Hills for evaluation. From behind a desk in a reception office that had the words "Intake Unit" on the wall, a pleasant woman took down all the insurance information and said the boy would have to stay for a few days to be fully evaluated. She promised he would be treated well. Saddened, embarrassed, but believing that some benefit would come of it, the Harrells watched their adopted boy being led through the door into the ward, and heard it lock behind him.

The next morning, after being unable to talk to Jason by phone the night before, Marianne showed up with a suitcase full of clothes. The intake clerk assured her that Jason was doing fine. He was "under evaluation," the clerk said. "Leave his things and we'll call you in a day or so. He cannot have visitors just yet."

The Harrells were concerned, but at least they knew where the boy was. Besides, Colonial Hills advertised copiously in the San Antonio area; its warm and fuzzy ads, with the slogan "Hugs, Not Drugs" above an 800 hot-line number, were familiar from television, from highway billboards, even from the backs of park benches. Colonial Hills was said to be the best. The Harrells relaxed and waited, figuring the boy was getting help.

This is where things stood late on the afternoon of April 12—the week after Jason was admitted—when the Sector One patrol car pulled up at the curb and caused Marianne Harrell and the four-teen-year-old Jeramy, who were standing outside, to turn around.

About a half hour earlier, Jeramy had come home from school carrying a stray cat. The cat was friendly and looked clean; Jeramy asked if he could keep it. His mother was in no mood to argue; she merely insisted that they take it over to the vet's to make sure it was all right, and that was where they were heading when the patrol car came up with its lights flashing, causing the cat to bolt out of the boy's arms and dart behind the garage.

The car was light blue, a four-door Dodge with a red light on top and the words "Sector One" in reflector letters across the trunk. The backseat was set up with a prisoner cage. Two hulking uni-

formed officers, one white and the other black, got out and walked
slowly toward the boy and his mother.

"Can I help you?" Marianne said uneasily, wondering what Jason
could have managed to do in a hospital that was serious enough to
bring the cops.

"Yes'm, you can," the white officer said, flashing a gold badge
on his shirt pocket under his coat, while the other planted himself
behind her son. "We're Sector One Mobile Crisis Unit, and we're
here to pick up the boy." The officer said his name was Lieutenant
Joe Saenz. At about six foot two and 220 pounds, he looked like a
nose tackle for the Cowboys, but the forty-six-year-old Saenz was,
in fact, a former guard at a state mental hospital. He was not, and
never had been, an actual police officer, although he had once been
licensed, for three months in 1986, as a deputy constable. Still,
Marianne Harrell thought he was a cop.

"He isn't here," Marianne said of Jason. "What'd he do?"

"*That* boy," Saenz said, pointing to Jeramy.

"What'd *he* do?"

Saenz allowed that he really couldn't say. All he knew was, the
boy had to come along.

Alarmed, but also feeling her anger rise, Marianne grabbed her
son by the arm, demanding, "What did you *do?*"

The boy protested shrilly, "Nothing. I didn't do nothing!"

The officers suggested they all go inside. There they found Sid
at the kitchen table, eating a pork chop.

"Put it down," his wife said. Seeing the two uniformed officers
tromping in through the living room behind her and Jeramy, Sid
paused in mid-bite. "There's something going on," she told him.

"What?"

"If you want the information on this case, you got to call Colonial
Hills," the black officer told him. "You probably got the number."

Saenz told the Harrells the boy was going with them one way
or another, voluntarily being best. "If he doesn't go for the twenty-

four hours, we get a warrant and he'll stay for twenty-eight days,"
he said.

"And he'll have a record?"

"And he'll have a record, yes."

Saenz had to go out to the car and make a call. When he was
gone, the black man, who appeared to be in his late twenties, gave
his name as Officer Ulysses Jones. Jones had been told the boy was
violent, but all he saw was a scared kid who wasn't posing any
trouble at all. Confidentially, he told Marianne that if it were up
to him, "I wouldn't touch this case with a ten-foot pole. But it isn't
up to me. We were called by Colonial Hills Hospital and told to
come and pick up Jeramy on orders of Dr. Bowlan."

"Who is Dr. Bowlan?" she wanted to know. The boy had never
seen anyone with that name.

Marianne furiously grabbed the phone and called the hospital.
Tapping her foot, she waited till she got a Miss Plunket on the
line. "What right do you have," Marianne demanded of Miss Plunket, "to send the police over here to my house to pick up my
child?"

Crisply, Miss Plunket replied that the proper papers had been
signed and that the officers were acting legally. "They were exe-
cuted today by Dr. Bowlan," she said, naming a man who was a
Colonial Hills psychiatrist. She also mentioned a child-welfare
agent whose name was on the application for detention. Marianne
had never heard of him either, nor was she aware that the man
had never in fact signed the paper. None of this mattered right
then, however. The boy had to come in.

"What for?" his mother demanded.

"Substance abuse," Miss Plunket finally said, "Plus truancy and
child abuse."

"That's a bunch of bullshit!" Marianne yelled, slamming down
the phone.

While she was on the phone, Marianne hadn't noticed that Jer-

amy had run outside, with Officer Jones right on his heels. The
boy would later tell his parents that he was afraid he was going to
cry, and he didn't want them to see that. He also wanted to see
if he could find the cat. Outside, Jones talked quietly with the boy.
Later, Jones would say that this was when Jeramy agreed to go
voluntarily to avoid trouble. But the boy insisted that the detention
sheet was wrong. He didn't use drugs, and his grandparents never
physically abused him.

In a minute, both officers came back in with Jeramy in tow. His
grandparents were horrified to see their grandson in handcuffs,
crying openly now.

Sid became incensed. Jeramy had never caused his grandparents
any major trouble. He was maybe a little cocky sometimes, but it
was always possible to get him right back in line. The boy's sole
goal in life was to enlist in the Navy and qualify as a SEAL, the
elite amphibious commando squad. To make the SEALs, Jeramy
knew, he had to keep his nose clean. He didn't smoke, he kept
himself in shape, he kept his grades up. Sid was certain the boy
had nothing to do with drugs, and he had never seen any sign that
he had any interest in alcohol.

Sid had supposed that Sector One was some kind of high-level
antidrug squad, something from the federal war on drugs that you
kept hearing about. But when he thought to look to see what kind
of weapons they carried, he was surprised that the officers did not
seem to have any.

"Just who are y'all, anyway?" Sid asked as they prepared to leave.

"We're Sector One," Saenz repeated. "With Colonial Hills."

"Where do you get the information that my son here is a drug
abuser?" Sid pressed them, narrowing his eyes.

"This is the diagnosis from the hospital," Saenz said. "They will
explain it to you down there."

"You don't mind if I call the Live Oak police then? Just to check
on the procedure? It don't sound right to me. You say the boy's a
drug abuser? Well, even if that's so, which I don't believe it is, he

belongs to the government, because I belong to the government. And if that's the case, why can't I take him on down to Fort Sam? Because they have got the best facilities in this town to check for drugs. Let me take him to Fort Sam and have him completely drug-tested."

"You can't do that," Jones said.

They took Jeramy out to the car while Sid was on the phone to the local police department. When Sid came outside, he found his boy already locked up in the backseat, inside the cage.

"Hey, ain't you going to wait for the police to get here?" the grandfather persisted. He and Marianne managed to stall the two officers on the front lawn until, with relief, they saw the dark blue Live Oak patrol car turn onto their block.

Warily, the Live Oak officer, Sergeant Anita Seamans, asked what the problem was. As Saenz and Jones stood silently by their car, Sid explained what little he understood about the situation.

"Wait here," the officer said. As she went over to confer with Saenz and Jones, Sid moved toward the Sector One car to give some comfort to his son. This caused the Live Oak officer to wheel around.

"Step back!" she ordered Sid in a tone that said he'd better. He did.

The Harrells couldn't make out exactly what the three uniformed officers were saying because of the radio squawking from the Live Oak patrol car idling in the drive. But it was clear the policewoman was insisting on an explanation. They saw her take some papers from Saenz and read them.

Then she brought the papers over to the Harrells and told them that her advice was to let the boy go with Sector One.

They weren't police officers, she explained evenly. They were licensed security guards with Sector One Mental Health Services, on a "pickup." They did have official-looking papers, including a legal "application," as yet unsigned by a magistrate, giving authority for an emergency apprehension of the boy. From one paper she read aloud that "patient is diagnosed as substance abusive, truant from school, failing grades, violent, aggressive, abusive grandparent, to where James F. Scott, from Child Protective Services, has been called in." Reading from the paper, which she referred to as "an application for emergency apprehension and detention," she said that "the applicant states that he/she has reason to believe, and does believe, that the risk of harm is imminent unless the above named [Jeramy Harrell] is immediately restrained, and that the applicant's beliefs are based upon specific, recent behavior, overt acts, attempts, or threats which are herein under specifically detailed." It was signed by Joe F. Saenz on April 12, 1991.

The policewoman folded the papers back up and said, "Mr. Harrell, since he is a minor, you technically don't have to let him go with them. But if you don't, they have the authority to obtain a warrant, which they would obtain immediately, and which would give Colonial Hills Hospital the right to hold him for up to twenty-eight days. The thing is, if you do let him go, he can be released in twenty-four hours. I suggest you let them take him. They already have him down for resisting arrest, and they can make a problem for him."

Astonished, Sid backed off and let the boy go. However, as the Sector One cops lumbered into their car, he shouted at them, "You better not give that boy no drugs! You better not put a needle in his arm!" Sector One waited for the Live Oak patrol car to clear out. Then, emergency lights flashing, they took the boy away.

The Colonial Hills psychiatrist, Dr. Mark Bowlan, had filled out an "inquiry call" sheet at 3:55 P.M. on April 12, ordering Sector One to pick the boy up at home. In the space marked "Problems/ Behaviors" Bowlan had specified: Substance abuse, brother claims physical abuse, truancy. He elaborated that Jeramy's brother Jason "said he had experienced physical abuse since grade school."

Bowlan also filled out an "Application for Temporary Commitment for Mental Illness" for Bexar County Probate Court, stating that Jeramy, the "proposed patient," was "likely to cause serious harm to self" and "will, if not treated, continue to suffer severe and abnormal mental, emotional or physical distress and will continue to experience deterioration of his/her ability to function independently and is unable to make a rational and informed decision as to whether or not to submit to treatment."

It was dark when the Sector One car with the boy in custody arrived at the magistrate's office, where the two officers had been told to meet their boss, John Blanks, who needed to bring them a completed application.

The office was not in the San Antonio familiar to visitors, the pretty city of backlit fountains and shops along canals, the buff-walled Alamo where the fierce independence of Texans had its finest hour. The magistrate's office was in the San Antonio of the other side of the tracks, in the shadow of the interstate, where a fourteen-year-old boy locked in a patrol car could glance out the window and see the brooding hulk of the city jail dominating the landscape, beyond a big illuminated billboard that read

**ONE-HOUR BAIL BONDS
OPEN 24 HOURS**

And another big sign that took up the wall of a building across the street and had a cartoon of a grinning Mexican wearing a sombrero and brandishing a big key:

A-AMIGO BAIL BONDS

And another, down the block:

ACTION BAIL BONDS: "YOU RING, WE SPRING!"

Waiting in the car for one of the officers to come back with the magistrate's signature on his paper, the boy wondered what was

33

going to happen to him. Two oversized men, jail guards, sauntered down the street to a tavern on the corner, the Jail House Café, which also had a sign out front. This one depicted a prisoner in a striped uniform haplessly looking out from behind bars, like the man in the Monopoly game.

In the seedy office, San Antonio municipal-court magistrate Quon D. Lew, unaware that the boy was waiting in the Sector One car outside, routinely signed the "warrant for emergency detention" certifying that the subject met all four criteria required by the state: 1. "evidences mental illness or is a chemically dependent person"; 2. "evidences a substantial risk of serious harm to self or others"; 3. "that the risk of harm is imminent unless the person is immediately restrained" and 4. "that necessary restraint cannot be accomplished without emergency detention."

Then, on the basis of some comments supposedly made by his brother, the boy was committed to a psychiatric hospital.

That first night, a Friday, the Harrells could not get any information on Jeramy from Colonial Hills. All weekend, the hospital stonewalled them, saying to call back Monday. Finally, on Monday morning, still unable to get a straight answer from the hospital, the Harrells' oldest boy, Rick, eighteen and determined to get to the bottom of this, got out the phone book, turned to the blue pages of government offices in the back, and began working his way down a list: police, courts, even the Army.

Finally, he got to the office of state senator Frank Tejeda, where the senator's savvy legislative aide, a young woman named Elaine Anaya, listened for a few minutes and decided that what she was hearing was important enough to call her boss out of a legislative session in Austin.

Tejeda, a bantamweight ex-Marine who made a statewide political reputation taking on corrupt judges as rookie senator in 1986, did not like what he heard. He decided to get the full story fast. On the drive back from Austin to his office in San Antonio the next day, Tejeda could have pointed out another sign that the Sector One car undoubtedly passed en route to the hospital with the Harrell boy that night. There are literally thousands of them along the state's highways, warning against littering, but also carrying unspecified, unmistakable implications about truth and justice in the Lone Star State. They say:

DON'T MESS WITH TEXAS

CHAPTER TWO

....

AMONG THE OCCUPANTS OF FRANK TEJEDA'S SENATE OFFICE, which was tucked in back of a shopping center off a highway near the Air Force base in San Antonio, was a gregarious parakeet named Pete that liked to flutter from desk to desk. When the front door opened, the bird would make a quick reconnaissance flight to investigate the activity. But during the week when Jeramy Harrell was in the hospital, there was so much commotion in Tejeda's office that the bird just wore itself out. By Wednesday, Pete wouldn't leave his cage in the side room.

Tejeda himself set the tone, hustling into the back office with staff members right behind when he got back from Austin.

"Maybe the kid is nuts," he told his assistant, Elaine Anaya, who followed him in with a notebook and some files. Tejeda was playing devil's advocate. "That's all we need, we get him out of the hospital and he goes and kills himself, or shoots his parents or something."

Tejeda had guts, but he also was familiar with the Law of Unintended Consequences. Right out of high school, for example, he had enlisted in the Marines, which meant he was in Vietnam before the ink dried on his diploma. There, he was one of the few nineteen-year-old sergeants in the corps; he was so highly regarded that he was headed for Officers Candidate School. Two weeks before he was scheduled to be transferred out in 1966, he caught a bullet in Chu Lai, and returned stateside with a Bronze Star, a Purple Heart, and a pretty good lesson about fate.

By 1991, a year into his second Senate term, with a master's in public administration from Harvard and a law degree from Yale on his wall, Tejeda was preparing to run for the U.S. Congress the following year. From the looks of it, he wasn't going to have to run too hard. The seat was vacant and Tejeda had made such a name for himself as a responsive politician that, so far at least, he was unopposed.

The civil-liberties implications of the Harrell case were enormously troubling to Tejeda, a wounded veteran who was himself the son of a wounded veteran, a Texan of Mexican-American ancestry. They don't come much more patriotic than that. Assuming that the initial reports were true, Jeramy's commitment was not only an outrage but a gross violation of constitutional rights. Furthermore, scare a kid like that and it never heals, he thought. Why not help Jeramy, why not run with the case, get some headlines, rack up some political insurance points?

However, an ambitious politician like Tejeda knew enough to consider the fact that even a prudent man can get careless and shoot himself in the foot. Anyone who has ever answered a telephone in a public office knows how quickly simple-sounding complaints of mistreatment can become snarled in contradictions. And worse, this was a sensitive area of mental health. What if the kid *did* pose an "imminent danger"? What if he grabbed a gun and turned it on himself or others?

Tejeda cracked the lawbooks, tracked down the regulations on involuntary commitment, traced the responsibilities of the state and county bureaucracies. Finally, he knew his instincts were right. He picked up the phone and explained the situation to an official with the state mental-health agency. "I want y'all to check this out," he said.

Meanwhile, his staff was making calls. Once they had talked to the Harrells and gotten Colonial Hills to confirm that the boy was detained there, they contacted the juvenile courts. Tejeda himself contacted the Board of Private Investigators in Austin and told them he wanted a report on Sector One.

The staff went over the Texas Mental Health Code and found, to their amazement, that the boy had initially been picked up without a valid warrant. The warrant was only obtained during the stop at the magistrate's office en route to Colonial Hills. Now the hospital was claiming it had the authority to keep the boy for continuing evaluation based on a diagnosis of drug abuse. Furthermore, Colonial Hills had bigger plans: A new diagnosis of child abuse had been assigned to Jeramy over the weekend. This meant that his parents could not even visit or call.

The mental-health agency got back with its report the next day. The case looked like an illegal detention. Furthermore, they had someone go to the hospital to take a look at Jeramy to see how "imminent" this "danger" was.

"Hey, Frank, this kid is okay," Tejeda was told. "He shouldn't be in that hospital. And another thing—"

"What's that?"

Other local private psychiatric hospitals were involved in questionable detentions, he was told. "This ain't the first time. That boy's experience isn't all that unusual." There were rumors all over the community-mental-health world of San Antonio: These hospitals even had school counselors on the payroll to supply them with kids. As word of Tejeda's interest spread through the community-mental-health grapevine, people began calling.

"I feel for the boy," one man said. "Something very similar to that happened to my son." Tejeda and his staff soon joined an informal network of people concerned about what was going on in these psychiatric hospitals. They spoke with parents, lawyers, cops, clerks who had heard intimations about similar tales, who were wondering, who knew somebody. . . .

The calls were coming from reasonable people with incredible tales of being abused, even kidnaped, by for-profit psychiatric hospitals. One of them was a man named Lewis Kyle Williams. Williams, a forty-one-year-old civilian carpenter at the Air Force base—who thus, Tejeda knew, was well insured under CHAMPUS—said he had been hauled off without warning by two men he initially assumed to be police officers, and taken against his will to a psychiatric hospital. A couple of things about Williams's complaint caught Tejeda's immediate attention. The man had been taken to Colonial Hills Hospital, which was the place now holding the Harrell boys. And the "officers" took him in an official-looking car with the name "Sector One" on the back.

When he told his story, Williams explained that a few days before he was taken away, he had been in a big argument with his wife—"not violent, verbal. I am not a violent man," he stressed. The police had arrived and taken a report. That, Williams thought, had been the end of that.

But a few days afterward, two physically imposing men—"pretty big boys," Williams said—pulled up in a Sector One car. The two men showed him a warrant for his detention, which stated that he posed an imminent danger to himself and others. "Much to my surprise, they took me into custody and hauled me away to Colonial Hills Hospital."

This was a Friday. By Monday, Williams was still unable to convince the hospital psychiatrist to let him out. In fact, he said, he was pressured to sign voluntary commitment papers "and make it easier on myself."

When he refused, he said, the Colonial Hills psychiatrist told him the hospital had scheduled a court hearing for his continued detention. The psychiatrist outlined the patient's dilemma thus, according to Williams:

"He said, 'Let me tell you a story. You are driving down the road and a policeman stops you and issues you a ticket for running a red light. You say you did not run that red light. You go to court and you're standing in front of the judge, and you say, 'Your Honor,

I did not run that light.' And the policeman stands up and says, 'Your Honor, Mr. Williams did run that light.' Now who do you think that judge is going to believe? Tomorrow, when we go to court, you're going to tell them, 'Your Honor, I do not belong in Colonial Hills, my wife railroaded me in here.' And I'm going to stand up and say, 'Your Honor, Mr. Williams belongs in Colonial Hills for one, two, three, four, five reasons.' Now who do you think that judge is going to believe?' "

Williams said he'd see. As it turned out, the judge believed Williams and set him free. The hospital bill was $4,500.

Meanwhile, as Tejeda's office dug into their case, the Harrells kept running into bureaucratic stone walls in their attempt to get their boys out. On Monday night, Sid had driven across town to Colonial Hills. At least this time (and probably, he thought, because they had had a call already from Tejeda's office) a nurse from the adolescent unit came out to listen to him.

But she was just as implacable as the others had been. "You're not allowed to see him," she said.

"What do you mean, I'm not allowed to see him? It's been over twenty-four hours. I'm here to pick up Jeramy and take him home."

The nurse's attitude was that the matter was not open to debate. "The orders are by Dr. Bowlan that you or your wife cannot talk to, cannot see or have any contact with your boys." The nurse did not show them, but the doctor's orders on Jeramy's chart were in fact quite explicit if somewhat ungrammatical: "Orders from M.D. is that Jeramy is not to receive visits from parents/grandparents."

On Wednesday, Sid Harrell called Tejeda's office to report that Colonial Hills had just told him that a county judge had signed a new order to detain Jeramy in the hospital. A few hours later, Sid called back. Now the hospital had another document: They had gotten the boy to sign a statement voluntarily committing himself for drug dependency. Harrell could barely speak through his anger.

Tejeda phoned the judge, Keith Burris, and asked him if it was true that he had ordered the boy detained.

Judge Burris needed only a second to consider his reply: "*What bullshit!*" he bellowed.

Within a few days, Senator Tejeda's astounded staff would tell Sid that Dr. Bowlan, the admitting psychiatrist, had based his diagnosis—that Jeramy abused drugs and suffered from child abuse—only on interviews of Jason. Bowlan, investigators would later discover, was practicing at Colonial Hills under a "temporary restricted license." (His license would be revoked by the Texas Board of Medical Examiners that summer after state officials filed charges against Bowlan for falsifying letters of recommendation submitted with his license application when he moved to Texas from Massachusetts.)

"This Dr. Bowlan, based on some supposed statements that were allegedly made by the Harrells' twelve-year-old [Jason], filled out an application, made a diagnosis. Sight unseen, never having spoken to the fourteen-year-old, Dr. Bowlan orders the fourteen-year-old [Jeramy] picked up and taken in!" said an incredulous and angry Tejeda. "The fourteen-year-old was taken in on the twelfth, and Dr. Bowlan did not see the fourteen-year-old, the one he had ordered in on an emergency, until the sixteenth."

Tejeda's office finally obtained a writ of habeas corpus and got Jeramy released on Thursday, after he had spent six nights in the mental hospital. Tejeda himself went to the hospital to take the boy out. *Even then*, with a state senator standing there with a court order in his hand, the hospital staff balked at letting the boy go. "I'm leaving with that boy if I have to kick the damn door down!" Tejeda said. The boy was released.

When they got Jeramy home, Sid and Marianne Harrell were deeply worried about his glassy stare and dragging gait, the results, they believed, of medication.

"They gave him some kind of drug, which we cannot find out

what it was," Sid would later tell state investigators. "They said it was to calm him down, make him sleep. We don't know what he had, but we do know that when we got him home, he was hell to hold. I mean, they gave him something that made him . . . it wasn't the same Jeramy that had left that house."

"It was a different boy when he come back home," Marianne added. "I mean, he was entirely different."

Jason was also released soon afterward.

And the bill arrived not long after.

"How much were you billed per day for each boy?" Sid Harrell was later asked.

Marianne took out the hospital bill, which numbered more than twenty pages. "Jeramy's bill runs around eleven thousand dollars for six days," she said, flipping through the pages. "Jason's runs around fifteen thousand dollars for two weeks." CHAMPUS paid the whole thing.

The experience left the Harrells shaken, not only because of the way they were treated but because they felt nagging guilt—somehow, they believed, they should have known better than to let Sector One take their boy. Sid began waking in the middle of the night and getting up to make sure the doors to the house were locked. Marianne Harrell thought often of her childhood. She grew up in Nazi Germany. The boys weren't as trusting as they once had been.

Neither was Frank Tejeda, now convinced that this wasn't a local problem. Discussing the Harrell case with colleagues in the halls of the state capitol in Austin, he began to pick up horror stories from all over Texas. Unauthorized detainments. People hauled off on false charges. Outrageous billing. Even rumors of "bounties" paid to counselors and community workers for delivering patients. Tejeda and others were soon shaking their heads in wonder at the Texas-sized audacity of it all.

Of the Harrell case, Tejeda said: "We found out that there were no court orders whatsoever. That child had indeed been picked up without a warrant." Colonial Hills records showed that on Wednesday, *two days after a state senator's office made its inquiry,* the hospital succeeded, just as Sid had said, in getting Jeramy to "sign himself in for chemical dependence." Obviously the hospital was trying to bolster its case for keeping him in. "But even though he did sign, this hospital had in their possession records—*their own tests*—that showed he was drug-free, that he was not chemically dependent, was not alcohol dependent. Yet they had him sign himself in as chemically dependent, after him being initially picked up without a warrant!"

When Tejeda's people looked at Jeramy Harrell's records, however, they saw that the diagnosis Dr. Bowlan had assigned to the boy on admission was post-traumatic stress disorder. And the counselor who examined Jeramy right after his admission (and days before Bowlan actually saw him) had written on his chart: "Jeramy says his brother Jason lied to get him in here, denies any drug use, says family does not abuse him."

As he hubbub grew, Tejeda later recalled, "we found that the Harrells' was not an isolated case at all. There were dozens of calls to my office, similar stories, some worse, some not as bad. But the common denominator was that these individuals all had insurance. Every one of them was covered by insurance." It was clear that this was a major scandal, and it stood to reason that if such things were happening in San Antonio, they were also happening in Houston and Dallas—hell, these hospitals were all over the country. Tejeda decided to move decisively but carefully, by the book.

At the Bexar County courthouse, there was a quick revocation of the emergency powers that had given John Wayne Blanks's Sector One the authority to execute, on behalf of private psychiatric hospitals, what Blanks himself now conceded were "warrantless detentions." Within weeks, Blanks's Sector One mobile-response business ground to a halt and he suspended operations. He called this a "damn shame," saying: "We feel that we have a responsibility to the mental-health community," he said.

Not long afterward, on a balmy spring evening when they might rather have been barbecuing in their San Antonio backyards, a group of locals, wondering what Frank was so riled about, crowded around the conference desk and folding tables that had been set up in the state senator's office. Tejeda had told them to be there: Steve Hilbig, the Bexar County district attorney; Dennis Mc-Knight, his chief of fraud investigations; Captain Jack Dean of the Texas Rangers; two judges; and a gaggle of sheriffs and chiefs of police, school principals and administrators—thirty people total, all of them gathered because they knew that someone had been misguided enough to Mess with Texas, and Frank Tejeda was fixing to do something about it.

Tejeda had charts. He had diagrams on a blackboard, which he rapped at with his pointer, like a member of an organized-crime task force going over the Mafia's hierarchy, except that these charts depicted the corporate organization of a psychiatric hospital and the interlocking responsibilities of the county mental-health and law-enforcement authorities.

He told them that Mrs. Harrell said that what had happened to Jeramy reminded her of her childhood in Stuttgart, Germany, during World War II, when neighbors were sometimes taken away by men in uniform without warning or explanation. Tejeda outlined what his staff had learned about the situation; he was blunt in his assessment of the problem. Illegal detentions were going on, and the problem wasn't just Sector One. In other illegal detentions, moonlighting cops were doing the job. "Big money is being made," he said. "Citizens are being deprived of their liberty by a profit-making venture." Fees of up to $450 apiece were being offered for the delivery of people, including kids like the Harrell boy, to psychiatric hospitals.

Travis County probate judge Guy Herman, who had driven down from Austin, said that he had heard of Sector One and knew how to describe what they were doing: "This security-guard service apparently is attempting to expand its business to our city and county. It's my understanding private hospitals are being asked to engage the services of this entity in exchange for a fee based on the successful delivery of a body with liquid assets or unexpended insurance benefits." The judge knew what this was: "In yesteryear, there was a place for bounty hunters in Texas. However, today this approach seems out of place."

Claire Korioth, the chairwoman of the state insurance board, had another term for it: body-snatching.

Blanks responded that such allegations were "totally unfounded."

But the commotion down in San Antonio got a few people at the capitol to remember some stories about psychiatric abuse that had come out a year earlier, when a subcommittee of the state House Committee on Human Services had actually first cracked open the lid on the situation during little-noticed hearings on "throwaway children." These were youths who had been in disputes with their parents; some ended up in private psychiatric hospitals, only to be dumped when their insurance benefits ran out. There were also allegations that hospitals and addiction clinics were soliciting runaway shelters for leads. The committee had put out an interim report recommending that the legislature investigate; it was ignored.

Tejeda dug out a copy of that report and went to see his good friend Senator Judith Zaffirini, a Democrat from Laredo who was chairman of the Health Services Subcommittee of the powerful Committee on Health and Human Services. Taking her aside, he said, "Judy, we've got a problem down in San Antonio, and I don't think it's just localized. Can I fax you some stuff?"

Zaffirini, a former journalist, was appalled by what she learned. She spoke with an aggressive young senator, Mike Moncrief, a Fort

Worth Democrat, who also sat on her committee. Moncrief, it turned out, had some knowledge of the psychiatric business, since every major U.S. operator of private psychiatric hospitals had built at least one facility in the booming Dallas–Forth Worth region during the 1980s. Moncrief himself served on the advisory board of one of those hospitals.

And Moncrief was already deeply suspicious. He had recently received in the mail, anonymously, a commercial newsletter from PIA Press, an in-house publications division of National Medical Enterprises, the California corporation that owned Colonial Hills as well as ten other psychiatric hospitals in Texas. The newsletter, distributed to family-counseling, mental-health, and substance-abuse professionals, including corporate employee-assistance counselors and the clergy, promoted a successful marketing technique called "Books As Hooks."

In a chatty style, the newsletter boasted that program directors had discovered that "our books and pamphlets have made a significant difference to their bottom line and brought in thousands of new clients to their programs. . . . The 'Books As Hooks' strategy is working successfully at client hospitals across the country." It offered a free kit with "a marketing plan, press releases, suggestions for seminars. . . ."

The newsletter Moncrief got was festooned with testimonials to the company's books as "useful marketing tools." On it, a "substance abuse program director" enthused: "We've been using these books for three years. They do help us fill the hospital." A "psychiatric program director" added: "PIA Press books are one of the most powerful marketing tools we have. . . . Our attendance increased by 110 percent."

The crassness of trafficking so gleefully in human misery stuck in Moncrief's craw. The promotional titles, for distribution to vulnerable people approaching an employee-assistance counselor or a supposedly objective crisis agency for help, covered a wide range of emotional travails that could be exploited with these "useful marketing tools," including addiction, family emergency, adolescent depression, and the death of a spouse. There were titles geared to women, gays, blacks, Hispanics, Native Americans, and young adults "in recovery."

The Human Services committee staff went to work. By the summer, hearings had been scheduled all over Texas. Moncrief, ultimately appointed to run them, had this to say: "I don't know where the trail is going to lead, but it appears that at bare minimum we have uncovered a national problem, and at the maximum it is international in scope. I am horrified. I think we are the first ones in the country to turn over the rock and see what is crawling out from underneath."

CHAPTER THREE

....

Linda was betrayed in a church.

In the summer of 1991, Linda, a forty-year-old executive secretary for a corporate lawyer in Dallas, took a minister aside after the regular Wednesday night singles social in the basement of a Methodist church in the Dallas suburbs. He was kind and understanding, and she opened up to him about her troubles, feeling great relief when he reassured her with a smile and a gentle pat on the arm. He said they could meet the next night for counseling. "I'll call you tomorrow night with my schedule," he told her.

As he had said he would, the minister phoned at nine-thirty the next night. After a brief exchange of pleasantries, he said: "What I'm suggesting is that you come on by and we discuss your situation with a crisis counselor who helps us out professionally. She happens to be here right now, just finishing up with another person. Could you come over tonight?"

Wary about the hour, but trusting the minister's judgment, Linda shrugged and said sure. When she arrived at the parish house a little before ten-thirty, the minister led her to his office, where he introduced a middle-aged woman named Patty, whom he described as a "certified social worker." Then he left the two women alone.

At first, Linda found Patty disarmingly sympathetic and decisively reassuring. But she also had a disquieting sense of being carefully maneuvered, as if she were talking to a particularly canny salesman. At last, the agenda became clear. "You know, I think you're suicidal," Patty said after they had been talking for forty-five minutes. "You need treatment." This blunt appraisal had its effect. Linda was quickly in tears; she became confused, defensive, and alarmed.

Suddenly, she knew this was more than a pastoral counseling session. She wondered where her minister was. "Are you talking about me going into a hospital?" she asked nervously. Watching her evenly, the counselor made it clear that the discussion had come to a conclusion.

"You are a danger to yourself," Patty replied, dropping all the cordiality. She told Linda she needed to be admitted immediately to Brookhaven Psychiatric Pavilion, which was one of six north Texas private psychiatric hospitals run by National Medical Enterprises. Hospitals like Brookhaven Psychiatric Pavilion were familiar names in the Dallas area because they advertised themselves relentlessly on television with warm-toned commercials that emphasized sympathetic understanding and a program of carefully designed medical treatment for depression, alcoholism, family crises, and many of the other stresses and tribulations of everyday life. The commercials always managed to project a soothing message quite unlike the harsh and authoritative one that Linda was hearing now in the church office. "We would much rather put you in a hospital than attend your funeral," the counselor told her in the tone of voice a parent might use to address a child who refused to go to school. "You are going in, tonight."

Linda tried to explain that she was mildly depressed, not suicidal, and certainly not crazy, but her protests had no effect at all. "You're a crisis counselor," she said, summoning as much indignation as she dared, "not a psychiatrist or a psychologist. A crisis counselor making a diagnosis!"

The counselor replied, "You leave me no choice. I'm exercising my authority. I will have you put in."

Feeling cornered and alone, Linda begged to make a phone call. It was now after midnight. The counselor left her alone in the office. Linda overheard the pastor on the line in the next room. She froze in horror when she heard him ask for an ambulance to respond to a psychiatric emergency.

"The most terrifying aspect of my encounter was that it took place in the dead of night," Linda would recall later. "The crisis counselor authoritatively stated that if I didn't voluntarily admit myself to several days of observation at Brookhaven, she would have a warrant issued for my arrest because she said I was a threat to myself."

Linda took the only way out: She fled. She ran out of the church as fast as she could, fumbled for her keys, got into her car, and sped away as if the hounds of hell were after her. It was the best decision she had made so far that night.

"I was frightened. Terrified. I was afraid to go home for fear that the police would be waiting to arrest me. I didn't know what to do or where to go," Linda said. She drove across town and pounded on the door of a friend's house until she woke her up. Inside, she ran to the phone. "I called all over Dallas—the police, crisis hot lines—just trying to sort this out, wondering what I could do to prevent this from happening to me." The advice she got was to find a lawyer. A lawyer, at one o'clock in the morning? Finally, she phoned the church, hoping desperately to be told that it had all been a terrible mistake. The crisis counselor picked up on the second ring.

"Where are you?" she demanded.

Linda couldn't speak.

"You *will* be put in," the counselor threatened.

Afraid that they could trace the call, Linda hung up and looked up the night number for the Brookhaven Hospital. She felt physically ill when the person she talked with recognized her name and said that Brookhaven had just obtained a detention warrant for her from a court. She dropped the phone as if it had just burst into flames.

Finally, at three-thirty A.M., she looked up the number of her boss, the lawyer. When he heard the name "Brookhaven" he woke right up. "Oh, my God," he said. "I know that place." By coincidence, a friend who was a community mental-health counselor had recently told him amazing stories about innocent and apparently fully rational people being detained involuntarily in private psychiatric hospitals desperate to fill beds with insured patients. And now here was his secretary, a woman he knew and respected, hysterical in the middle of the night, and it sounded as if exactly that was happening to her.

He settled Linda down and persuaded her to get some sleep. The next morning, she met with her boss's friend, who "called off the dogs," as she would put it later. But there had been no mistake; the county apparatus for dealing with psychiatric emergencies had indeed been put in motion in Linda's case. That meant that she now had to prove herself sane. Before it would agree to drop the application for a detention warrant—which would be routinely issued by a court—the hospital insisted that she undergo an independent psychiatric evaluation "to prove that I was not a danger to myself, suicidal or [clinically] depressed," Linda said. The psychologist who did the evaluation found no indication that Linda was suicidal, and was dumbfounded by the idea that anyone would want to put her in a psychiatric ward.

Like others who have publicly discussed their stories of abuse at the hands of profiteering psychiatric hospitals, Linda maintained that she was deeply mortified by the experience; an intimation of psychiatric illness is not something most people want lingering around their reputations. Still, she decided to "take a stand" and "offer support to others who have had similar horrifying experiences." She said she could not believe that this had happened to her, without warning, in the United States. "For almost twenty-four hours, beginning in the dead of night, I was terrified of being taken away," she said. "I was fortunate. I was not carted off in the middle of the night. But I will never forget the terror."

All across the country, others weren't so lucky. Here are some of their experiences.

Marital disputes often opened the way for psychiatric-hospital abuses, some of them involving very young children.

In 1987, Fair Oaks Hospital in Boca del Rey, Florida, told George Pallay that he couldn't take his three children—two daughters, ages nine and eight, and a son, three—out of the psychiatric ward, where they had been placed by their mother during a custody dispute. The father, whose health insurance provided liberal psychiatric benefits, was rebuffed repeatedly when he tried to have the children released.

The hospital was housed in a modern two-story building complex that resembled a corporate conference center and had a pond in front. It was one of the most heavily advertised private psychiatric hospitals in the affluent West Palm Beach region, an area that had three such facilities in 1985, and ten of them two years later, with the psychiatric hospital business at its peak of expansion. Fair Oaks, owned by NME, had a full-cover ad on the back of the local phone book that boasted of its full range of adult and adolescent psychiatric programs, including an on-site school.

A court-appointed guardian who visited the Pallay kids in the children's and adolescent psychiatric ward wrote: "The children may be upset and anxious, but they do not appear to be, according to anyone, psychotic or deviant, deserving institutionalization."

Pallay did manage to get his children out—after they had been in the hospital for over a month. A subsequent lawsuit contended that "none of the children were mentally ill, nor did they require locked confinement or restraint," and that they were ultimately released just twenty-four hours before the yearly mental-health-insurance maximum benefit ran out, "even though the insurer had advised the facility two weeks earlier that the confinement was medically unnecessary." The insurance company paid the $108,000 bill.

Pallay's suit was later settled.

Meanwhile at NME's Baywood Hospital in Webster, Texas, a lawsuit charged that a two-year-old was inappropriately detained for two weeks in 1991. The same lawsuit alleged that at Yorba Hills Hospital in Yorba Linda, California, a seven-year-old boy was hospitalized for three months for "depression psychosis."

In Alabama, a boy's foster parents ended up battling a psychiatric hospital for custody after they took him there for an evaluation.

"Larry and Patricia Barker are the foster parents of an eight-year-old boy named Daniel," recalled Curtis L. Decker, the director of the National Association of Protection and Advocacy Systems. NAPAS, based in Washington, is a nationwide patients'-rights group that began accumulating evidence of large numbers of abuse cases involving psychiatric hospitals in the early 1980s. "The Barkers were having a little difficulty toilet-training Daniel, and decided that some counseling for the boy might be of some help. What started out as a concern to help their foster child turned into a nightmare for the Barkers."

After an initial session, Daniel was removed from the custody of his foster parents and placed in a seven-month inpatient treatment program. The Barkers alleged that the boy was overmedicated and put in isolation, and that he became withdrawn and disturbed. "The Barkers were restricted from seeing Daniel to only specific and limited visiting hours. Only after the Barkers sought legal and political help was the boy returned to the family," said Decker.

At Acadian Oaks Hospital in Lafayette, Louisiana, a fourteen-year-old spent three months in the psycho ward in 1991 for what a lawsuit called "the relatively minor condition of 'adjustment disorder.' " At Laurelwood Hospital in Woodlands, Texas, insurance bills for a thirteen-year-old boy showed him participating in forty-one group-therapy sessions in one day. Had they taken place (and a lawsuit asserts they did not), the boy would have been in "around the clock therapy," as the complaint put it. At the same hospital, a psychiatrist made this notation on the discharge records of a five-year-old child, according to court documents filed in connection with a lawsuit: "He maximized his hospital benefits and aftercare plans were finalized."

In 1992, a man whose wife had stormed out on him opened the Yellow Pages to "Health Care" and found an 800 number that seemed to offer help for the couple's two teenaged children.

Since he lived near Albany, New York, the man was surprised when he learned that the 800 number was actually for a private psychiatric hospital in southern California. But the pitch was re-assuring: The hospital offered a comprehensive treatment program for kids whose parents were having marital difficulties. To a worried father in a snowbound upstate New York winter, southern California sounded like a glamorous place to send his daughter, sixteen, and son, fifteen, to be treated for adjustment difficulties while he and his wife battled over their marriage. It sounded like a resort. The hospital said the program even included trips to Disneyland. His wife's employee insurance benefits from G.E. would cover it all.

When the father agreed, the hospital's representative said that two plane tickets would be sent out immediately. The kids would be met at the Los Angeles airport by a hospital staff member who would have a code name: Santa Claus. The tickets arrived two days later by Federal Express: $695 apiece, one way.

"The kids got in at three-thirty in the morning," said their mother, who later reconciled with her husband, "and were im-mediately given legal papers to sign, including a form that said they agreed not to leave the hospital for at least ten days."

The next day, the woman, then staying with a relative, received a call from the hospital "saying that the kids needed me. They suggested that they could put me in the program, too."

She flew to California to join her children. The hospital had her sign the papers for all three of them. Admitted under a diagnosis, she said, of "co-dependency," she was placed in a locked psychiatric ward near the unit where her son and daughter also were being held. Though she had no medical problems, and had signed the admission form for herself because she was told it was the only way her children could be treated, the woman was given a series of tests, including expensive medical procedures, as were the kids.

Meanwhile, the children attended a few hours of classes each day and frequent sessions of group therapy. The boy, recalling his experiences later, said that he tried both crack cocaine and marijuana for the first time, thanks to other kids who smuggled it into the hospital. He was particularly impressed with the wide range of experiences and ages of his fellow patients, one of whom was a two-year-old accompanied by her mother.

He recalled one staff addiction counselor who himself was recently out of rehabilitation. "At dinner, if you talked too much, he would put you in the Time Out room." The main feature of the Time Out room was a flat bed with leather restraints.

"I didn't have a problem," said the mother. "Facing divorce is a big crisis, but you have to get through it on your own. But after that hospital, I was scared to come home."

The woman's insurance covered thirty days of inpatient psychiatric care for her and her children, and the hospital "cleaned the insurance company's clock," she said. Though her daughter insisted on leaving after three weeks, her son was kept an extra week, for a total of five.

However, the program had no virtue that she could see. "My son came back worse than ever, drinking, staying out later. He thought he was Mr. Cool. He told his friends he had been on vacation in California for five weeks."

Furthermore, she said, the promised "aftercare" program consisted of a list of phone numbers of welfare agencies.

Ironically, she found one that actually offered what she thought she and her children needed: good and honest counseling, without a hidden agenda. In 1993, she and her son were still going to weekly group sessions at the Catholic Family Community Mental Health Center, near their home. "They charge ten dollars a week," she said. "This is all any of us needed."

The victims of psychiatric profiteering include old people as well as young ones.

In Anniston, Alabama, W. T. Gable, a retired insurance agent, took his wife to Regional Medical Center in 1991 to have her treated for sleep disturbances brought on by a diabetic emergency. She ended up in the hospital's psychiatric unit, where, her husband charged, she was kept until her insurance benefits ran out twenty-eight days later. "I'd take my wife to the cemetery before I'd take her back there," Gable told the *Anniston Star*. A few months later, the hospital's only psychiatrist, William Nagler, was abruptly fired after nine months on the job. Nagler said he was dismissed because he had "completely refused to play their criminal policy. They said they've got to keep patients twenty-one to twenty-eight days, but it's not the job of some corporation to tell me when my patients should go home." He called the corporate policy "an absolute scam particularly designed to bleed patients' insurance."

In 1991, Major L. Harper, a seventy-four-year-old retired nursing home inspector from Fort Worth, Texas, took his wife, Jean, then sixty-nine and shaky after undergoing radiation therapy for cancer, to Psychiatric Institute of Fort Worth. The couple had been lured by the hospital's advertisements for a program to combat depression. But Harper was suspicious from the moment they arrived. "They were in a rush to get my wife admitted," he recalled, noting that the admissions staff appeared to be excessively interested in the Harpers' insurance coverage. For Harper, a man who likes to know exactly where the money is going even when someone else is paying the bill, this was a red flag.

At admission, he pressed for details. "Now, it's five hundred and seventy-five dollars a day for the room?" he said, amazed at the price. "What else?"

"Your insurance is going to take care of it," he was told.

"Well, I like to know the ins and outs," he said evenly.

From the first, Harper didn't care for the people to whom he was entrusting his wife. "They wouldn't meet you eye to eye," he said. And he felt they regarded his wife more like an "inmate" than a patient. For her sake, he kept quiet.

Still, he figured that at $575 a day for the room, she shouldn't have had to make her own bed, but she did. An initial "assessment" interview by a nurse cost $63, "and the room that she did the interview in, that cost us another thirty-seven dollars." Insisting on reviewing the bill periodically, Harper was flabbergasted by what he regarded as questionable charges: $108.59 for each "group therapy" session, sometimes four or five times a day . . . $65.75 for an inhaler . . . $62 for a Remington rechargeable razor that his wife never saw or needed . . . $4 each for diuretic pills that the neighborhood druggist told Harper that he bought at a hundred for $4 . . . $63 to talk to a "dietary consultant" and change a meal.

For a while, Harper held his tongue. But after his wife had been hospitalized for nearly a month, as her anxieties worsened with medication and the regimentation of psychiatric confinement, after she had lost twenty pounds and looked as if she was dying, as she pleaded for him to get her home, Harper decided he'd seen enough. He went to check her out.

They wouldn't let her go. In fact, the hospital threatened to get a court order to keep her in. This was the wrong thing to say to Major Harper.

"Court order?" he exploded. "You've done threatened the wrong person now. Don't you ever threaten me with a court order to keep my wife anywhere. It just ain't going to be done."

He took Jean home, where her condition improved rapidly. Meanwhile, Harper himself was ready for a straitjacket when he saw the bill, which totaled $38,714.18—including more than $5,000 for drugs.

Despite Harper's insistence that it was being ripped off, his insurance company paid the bill without a murmur.

Intensively advertised and nationally promoted by the news media, treatment programs for addictions and eating disorders offered ample opportunities for psychiatric hospitals to tap into the insurance coverage of teenaged girls.

Seventeen-year-old Kelly DeWald spent thirty-five days in Lake Hospital, an NME facility near West Palm Beach, Florida, for treatment of an eating disorder, in 1987. Actually, she said years later, it was her impression that she was there because of an eating disorder, though she couldn't find much evidence that the hospital actually had the specialized program of which she'd been told. Most of the treatment, she recalled, revolved around "Alcoholics Anonymous meetings, Narcotics Anonymous meetings, and viewing films and attending lectures on cocaine abuse and alcoholism," neither of which was a problem she had. She was, however, given a thirteen-page pamphlet on anorexia nervosa and a book called *Fit or Fat*. The hospital would later explain that anorexia is treated as an addiction, and patients share classes with substance abusers.

DeWald kept the itemized hospital bill, on which she had highlighted a number of charges:

- $17.50 for one Actifed tablet
- $750 for a Rorschach test
- $231 for 140 vitamin B tablets
- $532 for a thyroid test
- $504 for two urine tests for drugs

After she had been there for three weeks, DeWald said, a doctor put her on Pamelor (nortriptyline), an antidepressant that made her anxious and disoriented. (According to the manufacturer's profile of the drug, confusion and disorientation are the two possible side-effects.)

Six days after starting her drug regimen, the girl was given a battery of psychological tests (billed at $1,000) and told to forget the eating disorder. What she really had was "histrionic personality disorder," which would require four to five months more inpatient treatment.

Histrionic personality disorder, as clinically defined, covers a lot of territory. According to psychiatry's clinical bible, the *Diagnostic and Statistical Manual of Mental Disorders (DSM-III-R)*:

> *The essential feature of this disorder is a pervasive pattern of excessive emotionality and attention seeking . . . Their style of speech tends to be expressionistic and lacking in detail. For example, a person may describe his vacation as "Just fantastic," without being able to be more specific.*

By this point, Kelly DeWald and her parents were ready for a vacation—away from Lake Hospital. The DeWalds checked their daughter out. The bill was $22,500.

Another teenaged girl in Florida stayed in a psychiatric hospital for many months, diagnosed as having a "non-aggressive parent-child problem," when she became depressed after totaling her new car and gaining weight in 1986.

Both Traci Jo London, then sixteen years old, and her mother, Linda London Luca, had been impressed by advertisements from Fair Oaks Hospital in Delray Beach, promoting programs for adolescent stress and eating disorders. Traci remembered thinking, "Wow, this sounds great. This sounds like camp."

"I had a tremendous insurance policy from a very good job," her mother recalled. As it turned out, she needed it. Her daughter's stay at Fair Oaks was a lengthy one. "From March 24 until July 27, she was doing very well at the hospital," said the mother. "I visited her often, taking her out every weekend on a pass. She was going to school at the hospital. . . . She was elected president of the community and was a leader."

On July 16, home on a pass, expecting to be fully released in a week, Traci sank into a depression. She was taken back to the hospital, where her mother was told the girl was suffering from a fear of being released. The mother was more concerned about the heavy medication Traci was under.

"She was lethargic," said the mother. When she pressed Traci's doctor, "he told me that they knew what they were doing, that they were doctors and that it was a hospital where she was getting the finest care that she could possibly receive. And he assured me that she was getting better."

She did not. On July 27, the day after she returned to the hospital, Traci had what her mother called "a total breakdown. She did not know who she was. It was like she was on an LSD trip. . . . It was like she was four years old again—she totally reverted. She walked constantly; she was always on her feet, just pacing. I couldn't take her out [of the hospital] because I didn't know what was wrong with her."

Traci finally was discharged from Fair Oaks in November—eight months after being hospitalized, on the day her mother's insurance benefits for Traci reached their limit. Fair Oaks records diagnosed her as suffering from "atypical depression, non-aggressive parent-child problem, obesity, severe psychosocial stressors and poor adaptive functioning."

A clinical pharmacist hired by the girl's mother found that "powerful antipsychotic/antianxiety drugs in dosages beyond her tolerance" had been administered to Traci. After reviewing the medical records, the pharmacist, Mura Mathason, concluded that the girl "got progressively worse as a result of the treatment she received at Fair Oaks. . . ."

Single parents anxious about their children are avidly courted by the heavy advertising that characterizes the industry. In Texas, those who expressed worries that their children had been sexually abused or assaulted were especially vulnerable because of a state program that made financial grants available for the treatment of crime victims.

A young Texas mother named Victoria became concerned in the summer of 1991, when her little girl, eight years old, began showing signs of what Victoria thought might be the hyperactivity syndrome she had seen discussed frequently on television talk shows. The child was irritable and sometimes disruptive. Victoria wondered if she might have been abused in a day-care center.

This was when an ad in the local paper caught her attention. SET A NEW P.A.C.E FOR YOUR CHILD THIS SUMMER, the headline read. Next to it was a sketch of children happily roller-skating. P.A.C.E. was defined as "Problem-solving, Achieving, Coping and Encouraging" in the ad, which announced a "rewarding, therapeutic" outpatient program for young people with "emotional and/or behavioral problems." The summer program offered classes in math, English and science, as well as swimming, tennis, field trips, and "life skills training." The bottom of the ad was very encouraging: "P.A.C.E. welcomes kids ages 5 through 18 and is covered by most insurance."

Curious, Victoria phoned the number given in the ad and was told to bring her daughter to Bedford Meadows Hospital, near Fort Worth, for a free evaluation. According to Victoria, when she arrived a few days later, the first subject of discussion was insurance. Then the hospital evaluation counselor gave Victoria a form, explaining that because she had expressed fears that her daughter might have been sexually abused at the day-care center, the girl qualified for up to $25,000 in benefits under the Texas Crime Victims Compensation Act.

This sounded fine. However, she said, they began talking about putting her daughter in the hospital for observation, immediately. Frightened, the mother signed the admission form.

That was the last she saw of her daughter for four days. Denied visitation, Victoria became angry. At that point, she learned how quickly her options as a parent could narrow, once her child had been officially classified as a potential victim of abuse. When she protested, the hospital filed a report with the state department of human resources, reporting her as a potential child-abuse suspect. Victoria's innocent response to an ad had turned into a nightmare.

Next, counselors insisted that Victoria, too, needed psychiatric treatment—which would also be covered under the Crime Victims Compensation Fund. This wasn't a mere suggestion; Victoria said later that she was given the option of committing herself or being committed involuntarily.

A month later, mother and daughter were released. The bill was $30,971. "They put a price tag of $25,000 on my daughter," she said. "How could they do that?"

Another young mother told of having taken her four-year-old daughter to Texas's Laurelwood Hospital in October 1991 for an evaluation; she was apprehensive about emotional problems the child was exhibiting. A psychiatrist, suggesting that the girl might have been sexually abused by a male relative, ordered the child admitted on a "ninety-six-hour" evaluation, as provided by state law in such cases. The mother, confused and upset, went along when hospital staff advised her to sign herself in for ninety-six hours too, to "comfort" the child during her stay.

Five days later, resisting pressure to enroll in "drama therapy," the mother demanded that she and her daughter be released. Instead, she was forcibly placed in a straitjacket, given an injection, and confined to her ward. Two days later, the woman managed to call the local police in the hospital's Houston suburb. Police chief Joe Cantu already knew the drill, because this was the third false-imprisonment complaint against the hospital that he had dealt with in recent months. He made a call; soon afterward the mother and daughter were released.

In Fort Worth, a thirty-six-year-old mother recounted a similar story. She was worried in 1991 that her nine-year-old daughter had been sexually abused while the woman, an Army reservist, spent nearly a year on active duty during the call-up for the Persian Gulf war. Anxious about the time she had spent away from her daughter, she took the child to the Psychiatric Institute of Fort Worth for evaluation. Both mother and daughter found themselves imme-diately admitted to the hospital, unable to leave until relatives threatened to call the police.

"I was upset and very vulnerable. I said I needed help. I signed some papers but they didn't tell me what it was for," said the mother.

Crises such as the Gulf war presented ample opportunity for psychiatric hospitals to recruit patients among the well-insured groups of military spouses and dependents in regions near military installations. In Alexandria, Louisiana, NME's Briarwood Hospital distributed a pamphlet entitled "Coping with Crisis When a Loved One Is in the Persian Gulf." The pamphlet warns lonely spouses of the dangers of being home alone while a loved one is overseas: "Safety begins at home. Don't make it public knowledge that your spouse is away from home. . . . Contact the police or security force immediately if you detect any suspicious activity in your neigh-borhood. Above all, don't be afraid to seek help if you find yourself feeling overwhelmed." The pamphlet lists the hospital's toll-free telephone number for "a free and confidential assessment" and adds with measured reassurance: "We're here to provide support on the homefront."

In San Diego, California, the local affiliate of the National Association of Protection and Advocacy Systems, a federally funded psychiatric-patients'-rights group, found that during the buildup to the Gulf war, a sixteen-year-old boy was removed from class without his parents' knowledge and taken to a for-profit psychiatric hospital. A school counselor had reported concern that the boy, a high achiever, was "overextended" in extracurricular activities, with the added stress of an after-school job and a father who had been sent out of town for a couple of months to work on a military contract. Indeed, the boy had written a poem, one line of which read: "I can't take it anymore. Bang! Drop!!"

This caused him to be "evaluated," diagnosed as suicidal, and removed immediately to a psychiatric hospital, after which his mother was notified. Five days later, he was abruptly released—after the distraught mother convinced the hospital that the boy was not covered by CHAMPUS insurance since his father was a contract employee with the government, not a serviceman or military employee.

Any indication of emotional vulnerability could offer an opportunity for psychiatric profit. Two examples:

A Florida couple who went to a Tampa area hospital to attend a widely advertised "marriage therapy" weekend later claimed that when they tried to leave on Sunday, both husband and wife were separately prevented from checking out while hospital staff pressured each to sign papers involuntarily committing the other for alcohol abuse.

Meanwhile, a Florida man who did have an alcohol problem claimed that he was falsely imprisoned after he voluntarily checked in for a seventy-two-hour detoxification program. He charged that when the hospital learned that his insurance didn't cover alcohol treatment, he was rediagnosed with severe depression, which was covered, and was detained while hospital authorities sought a court order for his involuntary commitment.

• • •

In Texas, a man who hurt his back had a shocking experience when he sought treatment for pain.

"This can't happen in the United States. This *just can't happen*," said Charles Hagen, who went to a hospital for a back problem in the summer of 1991 and wound up against his will in a psychiatric hospital for ten days.

After injuring his back in 1988, Hagen, a forty-nine-year-old laborer from the scrub country of east Texas, underwent two years of extensive treatment, including visits to the Mayo Clinic, before a physician recommended a well-publicized pain-therapy program at Brookhaven Psychiatric Pavilion, a private psychiatric hospital in Dallas. He was assured that his health insurance would cover the costs for the program.

When Hagen checked in for the inpatient biofeedback program, he understood it would require a stay of one or two nights. But he soon found himself involved instead in intensive group therapy—and the talk was not about back pain, but about drug and alcohol addiction and childhood sexual abuse. Not able to understand what these had to do with his back, Hagen got impatient and said he wanted to go home. When they said he couldn't, he got very angry. Whereupon a doctor at the hospital diagnosed him as suicidal and obtained an order detaining him for "his own protection."

Informed by telephone that her husband had been placed on a twenty-four-hour suicide watch, Patti Hagen was horrified. "I remember saying, 'This can't be! He just has a bad back!' But the hospital employee stated that my husband was much worse than I realized."

Finally, and after being warned that they were acting against medical advice, Hagen's wife and mother hired a lawyer, who had to get a court order for his release. "They had done nothing for his back pain," said Patti Hagen. When Charles got home, she said, "It was like I was living with a stranger." Hagen himself likened the experience to "an Alfred Hitchcock plot."

• • •

For over a century, critics have charged that women have often suffered from a kind of tyranny from psychotherapy, maintaining that females are much more likely to be judged mentally ill and hospitalized for exhibiting certain behaviors—aggressiveness, guilt, sexual assertiveness—that are often overlooked in men. In 1970, a young psychologist named Phyllis Chesler attended a psychotherapists' convention and demanded one million dollars in reparations for women who had been "punitively labeled, overly tranquilized, sexually seduced while in treatment, hospitalized against their will, given shock therapy, lobotomized, and disliked as too 'aggressive.' " Chesler went on to write *Women and Madness*, a landmark in feminist philosophy that denounced psychiatry as intrinsically oppressive and antifeminist in nature. "Today," she wrote in 1972, "more women are seeking psychiatric help and being hospitalized than at any time in history." Around the time that was written, the private psychiatric industry was poised for the greatest growth spurt in its history.

For a woman battling severe depression, Mindy Jo Horvath had a remarkably sardonic view of life. From the moment she and her husband arrived at Willowbrook Hospital in Waxahachie, Texas, in August of 1991, she saw that looniness wasn't necessarily confined to the ward. During processing, she was told that her husband was "acting wild" in the lobby and would have to be admitted, too. "So I'm going, 'Oh my God, my whole family is falling apart,' " the thirty-four-year-old electronic technician recalled. But, it turned out, "it was somebody else's husband."

That episode set the tone for her twenty-eight days in the psychiatric hospital. "Basically, when I walked in the door, it was all downhill from there," she said. She had been admitted with the understanding that she would remain for a ten-day program. Her stay stretched beyond that and she was crowded into a ward with eighteen beds, some of them occupied by people who appeared to need medical treatment, not psychiatric care.

Like many other customers of the psychiatric-hospital business, she later read her bill with astonishment, thinking that if anyone needed a head doctor, it was her insurance company for paying all $32,538 without a peep. "One day I was charged for twelve hours of individual therapy, all in one day, at eighty dollars an hour," she said. "I may be crazy, but I'm not stupid." She picked up the phone and called her state senator's office to complain about the hospital's billing. She tried to put a light touch on her protest, focusing it on the absurdity of the experience. But it was difficult for her to wisecrack about the fear she felt day and night afterward. "I have no money left to seek professional help," she said quietly. "I was scared to death they were going to pick me up and send me back."

Even the most powerful professionals—doctors and lawyers— could be vulnerable to psychiatric-hospital abuses.

In 1990, forty-two-year-old Ronald L. Hedderich, M.D., was in his third postgraduate year of residency of anesthesiology at Southwest Medical Center, the University of Texas medical school in Dallas. At the time, Dr. Hedderich also was an anesthesiologist at Parkland Memorial Hospital.

His trouble stemmed from the fact that, as he conceded, he could be blunt and impatient in the operating room at Parkland. Specifically, it involved a dispute with a nurse over a misplaced fifteen-milligram vial of morphine ordered for an operation. According to a lawsuit filed by Hedderich, the nurse reported the morphine missing (it was soon found), and told her superiors that Hedderich's "behavior in the operating room either resulted from or was consistent with drug abuse."

The hospital's Impaired Physicians Committee intervened.

Though the committee had already been notified that the morphine had been located, Hedderich had to defend himself against an accusation of drug abuse. According to his lawsuit, two of the physicians on the committee "repeatedly confronted" Hedderich with accusations that he "was an opiate user and needed to come to grips with his problem by confessing his drug abuse to them, and by evaluation for opiate abuse" in a psychiatric hospital.

Hedderich saw this as an ultimatum: He could comply, or he could kiss his residency good-bye. He was told that if he wanted to keep his job, he was required to go to Brookhaven Psychiatric Pavilion and submit to drug testing and psychiatric evaluation.

Dr. Hedderich phoned his wife, Rhonda. Then another physician drove him to Brookhaven. There, the lawsuit noted, a psychiatrist's initial assessment stated that Hedderich's "judgment and insight appear to be fair." The psychiatrist left empty the blank on the admissions form for stating the reason for admission, though on the history and physical examination report, he did write "evaluation of the patient for possible substance abuse." The report also stated that Hedderich "was advised that he would have to be evaluated here or be removed from the anesthesiology program." For "further evaluation," it said, "he was admitted today to Unit D."

Hedderich was given urine and blood tests. Three hours later, a hospital physician called Hedderich's wife. "Rhonda, we have a strong suspicion that Ron has a drug problem," he said, mentioning the missing morphine, but failing to mention that, as Hedderich's wife had already learned, the morphine had at first been overlooked by a nurse and was found in a drug safe.

The next day, a hospital employee called to tell Rhonda Hedderich that the drug tests were all negative, but she was unable to obtain her husband's release. By now, both Hedderiches were also concerned that his confinement in a psychiatric hospital would cause problems for their ongoing attempts to adopt a child.

While at Brookhaven, Dr. Hedderich said he was forced to attend group-therapy sessions at which he was repeatedly asked to pledge himself to the quasi-religious principles of twelve-step programs. He was also told that any attempt to leave the hospital would be noted on his record as having taken place "against medical advice."

A psychiatric evaluation of Hedderich found no impairment, but used that assessment to recommend his continued treatment, asserting that since "there is no evidence of acute chemically based neurotoxicity," he would benefit from the hospital's program.

The report also noted the physician's denial (which, in the logic of intervention, is often considered a symptom of addiction): "Dr. Hedderich vehemently denies any current or past use of drugs of any kind . . ." His "noncooperative attitude" about completing a long-term treatment program was also noted.

A few days later, another medical report recommended continued inpatient treatment. Hedderich was also informed that a program of outpatient treatment would be required after his release from the hospital, and that his return to the anesthesiology residence program would proceed in tandem with the progress of his outpatient treatment, if he agreed to the terms. The Hedderiches, exasperated, called a lawyer.

The same day, Dr. Hedderich signed himself out of the hospital "against medical advice." His medical records indicated that his treatment had been not for drug abuse, but for a diagnosis of "adjustment disorder." His total bill for the hospital was nearly $9,000.

However, the lawsuit charged, although drug abuse had been totally ruled out, claims submitted by the hospital and its staff psychiatrists for treating Hedderich said that the principal diagnosis had "opioid abuse—unspec," with an additional diagnosis of "adj react—mixed emotion."

Dr. Hedderich returned to the residency program and subsequently found another job. He was stoic about what happened: "You can't undo it." He said he knows that he will have to explain himself in detail every time he applies for a job. "I'm still haunted by the horror of that experience."

The defendants in Dr. Hedderich's suit denied his allegations, and the case was later settled.

Larry L. Martin, a Dallas lawyer, and his thirty-five-year-old wife, Donna, who was hospitalized for three days in January of 1991 when she sought treatment for depression, also won't ever forget the ordeal.

"The events that occurred in the seventy-two hours to her, and similar abuses described by other victims, should be from a 1960 B movie, not reality at Baylor University Medical Center in Dallas, Texas, in 1991," Martin said. Through their experience, "my wife and I had our first true look at a mental-health-care system that is motivated by money and in which basic human rights guaranteed by the Constitution of the United States apparently do not exist."

When he and his wife arrived at the hospital, they both asked detailed questions about treatment and about patient rights and visiting hours. "The nurse explained that there would be no isolation. The nurse stated that my wife could receive visitors twelve hours a day. He explained that the staff would be warm and supporting. After these and a host of other promises and assurances, my wife signed in, and I left."

It was a decision they both quickly regretted. "I am convinced that this business is much like used-car sales," the lawyer said. "The objective is to obtain the signature on the dotted line. After the signature is obtained, the smiles are gone.

"My wife's belongings were taken from her. She was then placed in a large darkened room with no bedding or bathroom facilities. She was left there all alone, in the dark, all night, on a couch with no bedding. She was not allowed to use the restroom. In fact, because of this, she developed a bladder infection.

"No one bothered to tell her that her basic rights to communicate with the outside world by telephone or seeing anyone had been eliminated. The next morning, my wife discovered that she had no right to see anyone from the outside or to call anyone from the outside. When she was finally allowed to go to the bathroom, she was directed to the room of an elderly patient who struck her with a cane. She spent essentially the entire day in the same room.

"My wife was kept in the same room for all of the third day. She started her period, but was not given any feminine supplies. They

71

let her bleed on herself for hours. When she pressed to be allowed to change her clothes and clean herself up, she was threatened with being tied up in restraints."

Hospital records show this entry, made by a nurse:

> *Patient says, "I have to go to my room. I'm in my menstrual cycle, I have bled all over myself." Crying, wringing hands, depressed mood, remains restricted to day area.*

"They, a major hospital in Dallas, Texas, in 1991, asked me late Saturday night to bring feminine pads from my home to downtown Dallas, thirty miles away."

Martin continued, "As she bled on herself, my wife also witnessed what happened to another voluntary patient who tried to buck the system. This patient refused to be drugged. She was taken by two orderlies down the hall, pinned to a bed, her pants stripped from her, and forcibly injected with powerful drugs that left her in a zombielike state for hours.

"Throughout this time, the doctor was telling me to relax, trust him, that my wife needed time to adjust. He said that the hospital was an oasis for my wife, a peaceful, calm, safe place. He said that I should trust him. He would assert that the restrictions were necessary because my wife was being difficult. He seemed angry at her. He repeatedly emphasized that the hospital was an oasis.

"By the middle of the third day, the excuses were wearing very thin. I called to speak to my wife as her attorney. I was stunned when they refused to permit me to speak to her—yet another violation of Texas law. Within minutes, the doctor called and gave quite some song and dance about the importance of his rules and that he would not allow contact. He made it very clear that the medical relationship would be destroyed if I persisted and succeeded in contacting my wife. He said to wait until the next morning.

"The next day, I saw my wife for about twenty-some-odd minutes.

72

She was dirty, listless, she walked with her head down and her feet shuffled. She appeared drugged. She told me what she had been through. She talked of the shame and embarrassment of being left for hours to bleed on herself. As I left, I talked with one of the nurses and fished with the information Donna had given me. The nurse did not like these questions at all and emphasized that I should discount what my wife had told me."

What Martin had not been told was that his wife had been placed on suicide watch.

"I then contacted a friend who is a semi-retired professor at Southwestern Medical School. When he learned where my wife was, he told me not to believe them, that she might be drugged, and that I should get her out at once, using judicial contacts to get a writ if necessary. . . .

"I was forced to repeatedly threaten them. Meanwhile, the nurses were attempting to convince my wife not to talk with me. Finally, I spoke with her. I then went to the hospital and, as I stepped onto the floor, three nurses were by her side, talking intensely. As we spoke, there was a steady stream of nurses, always within earshot. I made my decision not to leave without my wife.

"I have never seen a human being reduced to the state that my wife was in when she got home. Later, she cried for hours as she explained what had happened to her. Psychological tests administered two days later showed that entire portions of her personality had stopped functioning, the result of the abuse that she had endured.

"Later, when I met with the hospital administrator and complained about isolating my wife in violation of state law and then abusing and neglecting her, the administrator laughed at my complaints about the illegal acts of the doctor, saying that it was apparent that I had never worked around a hospital because otherwise I would know what a doctor says is not questioned."

CHAPTER FOUR

....

BRENDA ROBERTS, A PERSONABLE COLLEGE STUDENT FROM Texas, wasn't aware of any of the industry's problems when she happily took a temporary marketing job during the Christmas season of 1990 at Willowbrook Hospital in Waxahachie. Bright and eager to learn as much as she could about business, she was proud to be a part of the hospital's hard-driving marketing team. "I'm a college student, I'll do anything," she said. "I mean, if I'm asked to go out on the street and sell Sprint, I'll do it."

To young people in Texas and other places where private psychiatric hospitals relentlessly promoted their services in recent years, places like Willowbrook are familiar adolescent reference points; an amazing number of kids say they know someone, often a friend or classmate, who has been in one. The way Brenda Roberts saw it, Willowbrook was clean and well-run; it treated the patients well, and the can-do spirit of the staff was contagious. In the staff lounge—where there was a big bulletin board on which the names of all the patients were posted, along with the names of their insurance companies and the dates on which their benefits expired—there was constant friendly chatter about new "contacts" and patient turnover.

Roberts would later testify about the relationship between insurance expiration and discharge date.

"Was there a large board in the staff rooms which was out of the view of the patients, showing the name of the patient as well as the insurance company and the date of the expiration of the insurance coverage?" Roberts was asked.

"There was a board in one of the units that had the name of the patients, the doctors, the expected date of discharge, and I assume that that was under the assumption of when that insurance was going to end. That's how many days we had to work with them."

"Was that on the board?"

"The expected date of release, yes, sir, was on the board."

"Was the date of the insurance completion on the board? In other words, the day the insurance ran out, was that also on the board?"

"I believe that the date of discharge was in conjunction with the date of the insurance."

As a marketing representative, Roberts mainly contacted area general hospitals and emergency clinics, where potential psychiatric customers—people who have had an accident, an overdose, a tragedy—can be found. She said she also maintained contacts with school counselors. However, contacts could be anywhere, "anyone you knew of . . . a potential patient that would need help, especially during the holiday season when, you know, people are alone and need someone to talk to." When Roberts talked to contacts, she told them about the programs at the hospital. "All I did was, I went out, handed them a calendar and a pen, said 'We're going to be here in case you run across anybody that needs help during the holidays.' "

Even for part-timers, there were bonuses for helping to keep the beds full during the Christmas holidays, a period when business in a psychiatric facility tends to be slow. Brenda herself won two tickets to a Dallas Cowboys game; her boss threw in ten dollars in cash—"popcorn money," she said.

Brenda Roberts was part of a trend. Like most other major entrepreneurial successes of the eighties, the for-profit psychiatric-hospital business was driven by brilliant marketing that did not miss any glimmer of opportunity to increase profits and market share and to devise new "product niches." To do so, it relied on thousands of community representatives and low-level crisis workers to bring in business, sometimes for much more than "popcorn money."

Until the marketing got out of control in the early nineties and psychiatric companies were forced to defend themselves against accusations of "bounty hunting" for patients, industry executives boasted openly and often of their prowess at beating the bushes for customers, wherever they might be found. Increasingly, the role of medical doctors—psychiatrists—in the admission of patients took a backseat to the role of "community referral sources": cops, teachers, crisis workers, members of the clergy, and corporate counselors.

Charter Medical Corp. is the largest U.S. operator of private psychiatric hospitals. In Charter's 1986 annual report, the company's president, William A. Fickling, Jr., stressed its intention of "being alert to new opportunities," and said: "We market our programs to referral services such as the court system and other legal sources, and to religious leaders in the communities we serve."

Clergy, with their access to people who have problems, are among the most avidly sought-after referral sources. A 1987 memo on employee marketing from an executive at Charter Winds Hospital, a Charter Medical facility in Athens, Georgia, offers employees cash bonuses and accumulated points for each tip that leads to an admission. At the end of the year, the employee with the most points would win a trip for two to the Bahamas. The memo also spells out the importance of getting referrals from churches: "Let me stress that clergymen are one of the most important referral sources that your hospital will have."

Schools, as Texas investigators discovered, also offered significant opportunities for market infiltration. In its 1991 annual report, National Medical Enterprises—which, with 6,300 beds and seventy-five hospitals, was then the second-largest owner of for-profit psychiatric hospitals in the country—boasted of its own interest in schoolchildren: "Many employees volunteer in the Adopt-a-School program, which NME supports and funds."

Indeed, throughout the eighties, the psychiatric-hospital industry was largely driven by marketing impulses rather than medical need. In its 1985 annual report, Community Psychiatric Centers (CPC), the fourth-largest player in the U.S. for-profit psychiatric industry, boasted that its extensive community-relations and marketing programs had become as important as doctors in generating business:

> *Approximately 50 percent of referrals to our hospitals now originate in the community so that, in addition to psychiatrists and other health professionals, referrals are frequently received from the clergy, school counselors and teachers, the judicial and law enforcement system, and from employee assistance programs maintained by many corporations.*

Routinely, psychiatric-hospital companies sent representatives to infiltrate Alcoholics Anonymous and other nonprofit recovery groups, and to approach networks of crisis counselors, employee-assistance representatives, hot-line workers, clergy, police officers, emergency-room aides, and even parole officers with rewards for delivering prospective patients who had potentially lucrative insurance coverage.

In California, a national toll-free suicide hot line, whose number is listed in phone directories all over America, has been characterized as a front for gathering leads on potential patients who had insurance providing mental-health benefits. The leads were in turn sold to local recruiters at private psychiatric hospitals.

Some of the for-profits' most egregious conduct involved children. To tap into the lucrative child and adolescent psychiatric market, hospital companies secretly enlisted school guidance counselors and others with access to student populations to identify and refer young patients.

"There are school counselors involved all over this state," Larry Bales, the assistant attorney general, told reporters soon after Senator Tejeda and other legislators began demanding answers in 1991. Texas authorities immediately subpoenaed the records of twenty-four school districts.

In many school districts, activity by recruiters for psychiatric hospitals was commonplace, and as aggresssive as that for college sports.

Hospital recruiters even lurked in the back of courtrooms to meet parents of teenagers having school problems and other difficulties. For years, judges have routinely sentenced certain miscreants to "counseling" and "therapy" programs, which often are run by for-profit concerns. In 1991, the potential for abuse inherent in such practices became clear when John Payton, a nineteen-year-old justice of the peace in Plano, Texas, near Dallas, began wondering why local psychiatric hospitals were so eager to provide assistance. Shortly after being named a justice of the peace, Payton had noticed that as parents of truants and other minor offenders left his courtroom with sons or daughters in tow, they were often waylaid by representatives of Brookhaven Psychiatric Pavilion. The "counselors" for this private psychiatric hospital, which had opened in a nearby town in 1987, diligently sat through hours of truancy hearings in Payton's court each week. The young justice's gasket blew when he learned that one seventeen-year-old high school truant left his court and ended up spending three weeks in the psychiatric hospital—diagnosed as suicidal—after Payton had merely ordered him to attend a free counseling session as his sentence.

"They were forcing these kids to sign themselves in," Payton recalled. He even looked up the standard diagnosis most often used, "bipolar disorder," which is psychiatry's current clinical catchall for various behaviors associated with degrees of manic-depression. "Because they're truant, they're manic-depressive," he said. A school-district official in nearby Dallas admitted that psychiatric recruiters also attended most truancy hearings there, but defended the practice as a way for "dysfunctional families" to get help.

Elsewhere, officials in the San Antonio school district were startled to be told that "intervention specialists" for Afton Oaks, a private psychiatric hospital owned by Community Psychiatric Centers, had routinely been given access to the records of the district's 62,000 students. In the 1990–1991 school year, these recruiters conducted "drug awareness" programs and held more than nine hundred individual counseling sessions with students. The school district provided office space and clerical staff for the recruiters.

Thomas C. Lopez, a San Antonio school-district trustee, received numerous complaints from parents that the hospital had pressured them to have their children admitted. Lopez went public at a school-board meeting in 1991. He denounced the "open season" on confidential information concerning students. "The public trust has been eroded," he said in a letter concerning the practice. "Every student's record and/or confidence has been available to a pair of intervention specialists from a for-profit psychiatric hospital without the appropriate releases." After Lopez complained, the school district suspended its contract with Afton Oaks.

Once marketing was established as the prime force behind psychiatric hospitalization, it was inevitable that obvious patient sources like Alcoholics Anonymous and employee-assistance programs, known as EAPs, would be open to manipulation. EAPs— in-house counseling offices to assist employees with addiction and other problems of interest to psychiatric hospitals—proliferated during the eighties. By the end of the decade, there were twenty thousand of them, covering more than one-third of all U.S. workers.

Envisioned as a progressive management tool to address the work-place costs of addiction and other behavioral problems, EAPs naturally collected pools of perfect candidates for psychiatric hospital solicitation—employees who confidentially approached their EAP were by definition already motivated (sometimes by the threat of dismissal) to seek help, and well-insured besides. All across the country, EAP representatives got to know the marketing specialists from private psychiatric hospitals; routinely, EAP offices are stocked with "educational" material supplied by such hospitals. And sometimes—it is a mystery how often—money has been exchanged. While the payment of referral fees is illegal in most states, and is strictly prohibited by most professional codes, it was an industrywide practice, investigators claim.

In late 1991 the *Houston Chronicle* noted the sharp annual increases in substance-abuse costs to employers and the corresponding increase in the number of company-run EAPs. The newspaper quoted the director of one private employee-assistance organization who said that some EAP officials received as much as $1,800 for referring patients to a hospital or treatment facility. Such payments were not confined to Texas. "Since the late 1970s, hospitals and treatment facilities have paid bounties for patients throughout the country," the newspaper was told by an official of the Employee Assistance Professional Association, a national group. The official said that the majority of EAPs did not take such payments, however.

Addiction counselors were also popular sources of referrals. In Texas, investigators learned of a psychiatric hospital conducting a seminar for sixty drug-abuse and alcohol-abuse counselors, most of whom are themselves former addicts, offering them the opportunity to boost their salaries from an average $23,000 a year to as much as $50,000 if they did what are called interventions and thus brought new patients in.

In Harris County, Texas, the *Houston Chronicle* found that doctors, counselors, court probation workers, and others who routinely encounter troubled people said they were offered bounties that ranged up to $3,000 for each patient they helped to admit to a local psychiatric hospital.

The pipeline from one Harris County court every month produced about eight hundred defendants facing charges such as drunk driving or drug use. They were evaluated by "crisis teams" from corporate-owned psychiatric hospitals in the Houston area. In some cases, the "evaluation" consisted of little more than a determination of the defendant's insurance coverage. According to the *Houston Chronicle*, two of the hospitals contributed to the judge's annual office golf tournament charity fund-raisers. Said a former recruiter from one of those hospitals: "The judge would agree to our recommendations and order the probationer into our hospital nine out of ten times." Another former recruiter said that hospitals routinely had pizzas delivered free to police departments and hospital emergency-room staffs to encourage referral of potential patients.

According to the newspaper, one Harris County probation officer bragged of receiving bounties for delivering ex-convicts to a private psychiatric hospital. The financial incentive was clear. In 1990 alone, Harris County spent $7.2 million to purchase from private psychiatric hospitals substance-abuse and psychiatric treatment, mostly inpatient, for people on parole.

Nationwide, psychiatric hospitals routinely cultivated such sources with free lunches and other favors. In some towns, private psychiatric hospitals arranged nightly deliveries of cookies and snacks to police departments and emergency rooms. According to the *Houston Chronicle*, one county probation officer who was paid $40,000 at his regular job had a second job moonlighting as a security guard at a private psychiatric hospital. There, he received two weekly checks—one for his part-time hourly salary as a guard and the other for delivering patients, with a certain amount each week for how long they stayed in the hospital. "They buy you drinks and then take you out to lunch," one former probation officer said, explaining how the hospital recruited bounty hunters. "They'll ask you to go on private hunting trips. You develop a relationship with them."

Until she blew the whistle, Janet Grigsby was the director of community relations and admissions for Dallas's Green Oaks Hospital, a psychiatric hospital owned by Healthcare International, the fifth-largest U.S. operator. In general, she was proud of the quality of the treatment offered at her hospital. But in 1987, shortly after being approached by a newly hired staff member who wanted to know more about the "Healthcare Network Referral System" program, she became troubled by ethical questions.

The program was spelled out in detail in a three-page memo from Healthcare International, but both the new employee and Grigsby thought the terms sounded questionable, especially the part about a $250 "incentive bonus" for facilitating referrals. The memo described the bonus as "a means of saying 'thank you' " for helping to process a referral or "a potential admission."

The new employee, an addiction coordinator whose job consisted mainly of helping to run and market outpatient programs, also was concerned about a letter from the hospital administrator confirming her employment. It described the bonuses available for helping to generate admissions: $200 for each in-patient referral, once the length of stay exceeded 14 days, and $200 for each "subsequent 14-day period in which they stay at Green Oaks."

After Grigsby raised objections, the hospital administrator revised the terms, to provide incentives up to $1,000 per month for total inpatient days. But no matter how she read it, the money was keyed to admitting patients. In February of 1988, Janet Grigsby resigned.

Another woman executive quit in disgust in 1990 after six weeks as a unit director at Laurelwood Hospital, one of NME's dozen psychiatric hospitals in Texas. The woman was earning $42,000 a year and was eligible for a $10,000 bonus for maintaining patient census levels. She said that she was ordered to do "whatever was necessary" to keep patients from checking out over slack times, such as the Christmas holidays, a claim that PIA labeled "patently absurd."

"All discharges were planned down to the day," she said. "We would look at the amount of insurance money. Say a patient had twenty-five thousand dollars in insurance and say we charge a thousand a day. We would keep him for twenty-five days.

"They had an obsession with marketing," the woman said of the hospital's management. This was one thing for the business side, but quite another when the physicians and other medical professionals on the staff were expected to share the same attitude, she said.

For her, the final straw came when, she says, her boss told her to "hang out at emergency rooms" after work, to make contact with the acute-care doctors, nurses, and admissions personnel who might be useful in referring patients for psychiatric care after their emergency. PIA strongly denied that allegation as well.

Of Lake Hospital in Lake Worth, Florida, a former staff member named Vicki Richards recalled, "Say they had six months of benefits, or fifty-thousand dollars or a hundred thousand dollars in benefits. They would stretch that person out as absolutely long as they possibly could to keep them there until the money ran out."

In 1988, NME was known within the industry as the "McDonald's of psychiatric care" for its aggressive market expansions. Even though bed capacity had increased by 75 percent in just three years, NME's sixty-two psychiatric hospitals, humming with an enviable 81 percent occupancy rate of their 4,900 beds, now accounted for about half of the company's overall operating profit. The man of the year was Norman A. Zober, the hard-driving president of NME's psychiatric-hospital division, and Zober saw nothing but good times ahead.

In the company's 1988 annual report, Zober expressed enthusiasm about NME's ability to meet the growing demand, as more employee health plans began offering inpatient addiction and psychiatric coverage and more firms set up employee-assistance programs to "identify and refer troubled patients." Zober noted that twenty-five states already required health insurance plans to cover psychiatric and addiction care, and that similar laws were pending in thirteen additional states.

Furthermore, he said, adolescent drug use was growing, "and stress in the workplace is so prevalent it is the subject of national magazine cover stories." Marital problems were on the rise, "and depression has been identified as a life-threatening illness," he said. Also on growth curves, he explained, were teenaged suicides, eating disorders, and various "debilitating character disorders and phobias" for which treatment was available at NME hospitals.

In terms that indicated no worry that the growth was about to slow, Zober boasted of NME's "satisfied referral sources" and of NME hospitals' success in handling what he called the "treatment-resistant patient."

By the end of the decade, however, psychiatric costs were rising so rapidly that U.S. corporate managers tried to put the brakes on by cutting back on lengths of stay.

Ever resourceful, displaying a flexibility and savviness that would have been more appropriate if applied to products such as beer or hotel rooms, some psychiatric companies promptly discovered a whole new niche market to help make up for the cutbacks: alcoholics and drug addicts from Canada.

Canadians pride themselves on a national health-care system that blends public funding with decentralized private delivery of services and that is responsive to public criticism. In the late 1980s, with the prophets of the Recovery Era protesting Canada's long-standing restrictions on expansion of psychiatric beds, Canadian officials decided to, essentially, subcontract inpatient substance-abuse care to U.S. psychiatric hospitals. The province of Ontario, with a population of more than nine million, offered the highest reimbursement rates, up to $1,500 a day for some patients to be treated in U.S. psychiatric facilities.

Anxious to keep their beds filled, recruiters from U.S. hospitals descended on Canada. One major U.S. hospital chain kept bounty hunters so busy recruiting alcoholics and drug addicts from the Canadian health system that it negotiated volume discounts with airlines to fly patients to the States. U.S. immigration officials found that during 1990, an average of three hundred patients a month were being flown out of Toronto's airport by U.S. psychiatric hospitals.

By 1990, according to Dr. Robert McMillan, director of the insurance division of the province's Ministry of Health, "there were at least several dozen patient brokers" operating in Ontario alone to funnel Canadians to private psychiatric hospitals in Texas, Florida, California, and elsewhere. "Bounties as high as $1,500 per patient were not uncommon before October 1, 1991," when Ontario sharply curtailed its payments after Texas authorities began investigating abuses in corporate-owned psychiatric hospitals.

McMillan's figures for the total expenditures show how successful those bounty hunters were. Between 1987 and 1991, the heyday of growth for the psychiatric industry, U.S. for-profit psychiatric hospitals collected more than $160 million from the Ontario government for providing substance-abuse treatment and other treatment for Canadian citizens. This compared with $17.5 million in the preceding five-year period. In 1989, Ontario paid an average of $18,800 for each patient treated in U.S. hospitals. One Canadian patient was nicknamed the "half-million-dollar man" by the Canadian Broadcast Company, which publicized a $438,000 bill Ontario paid for his twenty months of treatment in several private psychiatric hospitals in the Houston area.

To harvest this foreign wealth, bounty hunters for U.S. psychiatric hospitals worked, often furtively, throughout Canada to identify potential patients, including criminal drug addicts, who had national insurance benefits that could be tapped.

But much of the effort was aggressively open. On a downtown Toronto street, an electric billboard flashed a message: "Do You Have a Drug Problem?" The accompanying phone number was serviced by a company that received payments for delivering patients to psychiatric hospitals in the United States. In all, more than a dozen "referral centers" in Toronto were found to have contracts with U.S. psychiatric hospitals.

As they did with American patients, the U.S. hospitals often kept the Canadians until their insurance limits were reached, then showed them the ward door. Investigators who began looking into the situation in 1991 found that discharged Canadian patients were routinely dumped at airports without return fare, even without notice to their families.

Hospitals in warm states like Florida were especially adept at drawing Canadian patients. Dennis Jones, the administrator of Hospital Corporation of America's West Lake Hospital in central Florida, boasted to the *Orlando Sentinel* in early 1991 of the steady stream of new patients he was supplying on regular recruiting trips to Canada. "Canada made the decision several years ago to limit the number of psychiatric and substance-abuse beds," he said. "What they have discovered is that they made an error."

At Fair Oaks Hospital, the NME facility near Palm Beach, Florida, Canadian heroin addicts made up the majority of patients in the dual-diagnosis unit, where treatment was based on a primary diagnosis, such as addiction, and a secondary one, such as adjustment disorder. In late 1991, a month after the province of Ontario sharply curtailed payments for treatment in U.S. psychiatric hospitals, the occupancy rate at the hospital dropped by half.

CHAPTER FIVE

....

MIKE NICHOLS'S CLASSIC 1967 MOVIE *THE GRADUATE* HAS A memorable cocktail-party scene in which a middle-aged man takes aside the impressionable young Ben Braddock to confide the business opportunity of the future in a single word: "Plastics."

In the second half of the 1980s, the same kind of scene was playing within the close-knit business world of the psychiatric hospital. The word that was whispered? "Kids."

That was the time when the industry's movers and shakers, after their amazing burst of expanion in the late seventies and early eighties, took a moment to catch their breath and cast a hungry eye around. By 1991, the Big Four companies in the industry—Charter, NME, CPC, and HCA—would account for nearly 70 percent of the for-profit psychiatric beds in America. Competition for market share was ferocious, ever more so because a lot of corporate health-insurance providers were starting to get anxious about the staggering sums of money going out the door for what some suspicious employee-benefit managers regarded as Recovery Era palliates and $30,000-a-month "rest cures."

Here and there, benefit plans were cutting back a bit on the number of days of psychiatric hospitalization that would be covered. It was nothing major, nothing to get excited about, but in an industry that watched insurance-reimbursement indicators with the unblinking hawk-eyed intensity of global currency speculators, a vague sense of unease slowly settled. With so much new construction still on the drawing boards, the imperative was clear: New business would have to be found to ensure the double-digit profit-growth rates stockholders had come to expect.

In an interview with the trade publication *Advertising Age*, one marketing executive identified the trend in the mid-eighties when he declared: "There's a new market out there in grammar and high school–aged kids."

Pure economics explains the psychiatric hospitals' inordinate interest in children. The profit margin for a psychiatric bed occupied by an adult is 20 percent. For a child, it's 30 percent, since children demand less service and attention.

Within a few years, the frenzy to find kids with insurance and put them in psychiatric hospitals had become so overheated that one school official in California likened it to *Invasion of the Body Snatchers*. In the Arlington, Texas, school district, Madeline Taylor, the director of the district's secondary counseling and testing programs, recalled: "We were being besieged with people wanting to get on campus and get to the kids."

Some school officials, despairing at the lack of public attention being paid to the shanghaiing of children, believed that there was no way to keep up with the psychiatric hustlers. You'd shut down one hole and they were in another. In Los Angeles, Barbara Demming Lurie, director of the patients'-rights office of the county health department, recalled what happened when regional insurance companies, aghast at soaring costs for psychiatric hospitalization of children, began balking at paying claims for vaguely defined "behavior disorders." Abruptly, new mental illnesses were classified as the psychiatric diagnoses changed to pass muster with insurance companies. "All of a sudden, we saw an epidemic of major depression cases."

Profit-making psychiatric hospitals had run a brisk trade in adolescents since the introduction in the 1960s of federal Medicaid insurance, which poured tens of millions of dollars a year into treatment programs for low-income youths. By the mid-seventies, a series of court decisions had removed much of the legal authority that had long been used to commit troublesome kids to reform schools for noncriminal behavior, such as running away from home. Many of those teenagers—including a growing number whose parents had health insurance—became patients in for-profit psychiatric hospitals and on the psychiatric wards of about two thousand general hospitals. Increasingly, they were hospitalized under newly fashioned psychiatric diagnoses that provided clinical labels for a wide range of problem behavior. In some cases, such behavior (and kids of such a social class) had fallen under the purview of "reform schools" in the past. But increasingly, the behavior, and the kids, were the kind that would formerly have been dealt with at home, by parents, as part of the normal tribulations of child-raising.

Parental influence has always been a strong lobbying force in mental health. One of the leading interest groups pressing for more insurance coverage for psychiatric hospitalization of young people is the 100,000-member National Alliance for the Mentally Ill (NAMI), an organization representing family members, mostly parents, of people who have received psychiatric treatment. Estimates are that at least half of the seriously mentally ill people in the U.S. live with their parents, who shoulder many of the emotional and financial burdens associated with chronic mental illness.

Yet private psychiatric hospitals have no interest in the severely mentally ill, once their yearly or lifetime insurance limits are exhausted. While NAMI has been a forceful lobby for more funding for long-term treatment, its critics charge that the group has been coopted by hospital and drug money, and has become one of the most influential grassroots lobbies for the biopsychiatric-industrial complex in its push to have more forms of behavior classified—and covered by insurance—as mental illness.

Vociferous in response to criticism of biopsychiatry, NAMI is also closely aligned with the National Institute of Mental Health (NIMH), the federal agency in charge of U.S. mental-health policy and research. NIMH's main philosophical thrust is the buttressing of theories about biological and genetic causes for psychological disorders. This now-dominant branch of psychiatry considers itself a hard science and has close ties to hospitals and drug manufacturers. Psychiatrist Peter Breggin, a leading critic of NAMI, claims that the organization "pushes drugs the way the NRA promotes guns."

But by and large, NAMI represents families who have been regular consumers of psychiatric services. By the 1980s, the hard-driving psychiatric business was intently developing fresh markets, attempting to lure young patients to innovative treatments based on new, scientific-sounding diagnoses that had turned the profession of psychiatry inside out.

In trolling for more affluent children and adolescents, psychiatric hospitals cleverly used advertising and the media to exploit parental concerns about drug and alcohol abuse, as well as eating disorders, poor school performance, sexual problems, social stress, family crises, and even normal adolescent sulkiness and alienation. Many times, advertising subtly blames the adolescent as the source of a family problem. Almost always, the ads stress the peace of mind a parent can obtain by getting a child into treatment.

In a strictly business sense, the marketplace responded spectacularly. Between 1980 and 1987, the number of Americans aged ten to nineteen who spent time in psychiatric hospitals rose by 43 percent, according to the survey and analysis branch of the federal Substance Abuse and Mental Health Services Administration. In 1983, one out of every four patients treated at HCA's psychiatric hospitals around the country was a child or adolescent. By 1986, according to the company, the figure was one out of two.

Under industry prodding, the federal agency stopped counting adolescent admissions as a discrete category in 1987. Given general public concerns, the for-profit psychiatric industry clearly has no good reason to publicize the sharp increases in the number of young people admitted each year since 1987. The federal mental-health bureaucracy—which keeps at its fingertips remarkably precise statistics purporting to show how many children need treatment for depression, for example—isn't able to say for sure how many have been sent to psychiatric hospitals since 1986.

Perhaps coincidentally, the mid-eighties was the time in which the private-psychiatric-hospital business was near its peak of expansion, and moving aggressively to increase individual admissions as average lengths of stay stopped rising and the need to fill new beds became acute. Of the Big Four psychiatric operators, Charter opened twelve psychiatric hospitals in 1987 and HCA opened eleven; NME psychiatric hospitals' total capacity increased by over 50 percent; CPC's bed capacity doubled from 1985 levels.

Experts who study youth admissions now estimate that well over 300,000 adolescents and children each year are placed in psychiatric hospitals and treatment centers, both private and public, and that the numbers are still growing, especially among young children. One recent industry survey indicated that between 1989 and 1990 the number of admissions of children under thirteen increased by nearly 25 percent.

Few young people need to be hospitalized for their adjustment problems, these same authorities maintain. Indeed, a federal review in 1990 of five hundred psychiatric inpatient cases, most of them involving adolescents and children, found that two thirds of the hospitalizations were unnecessary.

Virtually all psychiatric inpatients are admitted only on the basis of a diagnosis by a psychiatrist or other physician. Defined with an eye toward insurance reimbursement criteria, whole new niches of problem behavior were added to the clinical purview of psychiatry; hospitals devised inpatient programs for new service areas such as sexual dysfunction and eating disorders. As new psychiatric hospitals opened their doors by the hundreds during the eighties, they ushered in a population of children with behavior problems that had never before been considered serious enough to require medical intervention, let alone hospitalization. In 1989, according to one industry survey, more than a third of child and adolescent inpatient stays were based on diagnoses of "conduct disorder," "adolescent adjustment disorder," and "oppositional defiant disorder."

At the University of Minnesota in 1982, a mild-mannered social-policy researcher named Ira M. Schwartz was perusing some state mental-health statistics while researching ways to shore up crucial social services for youths against the wholesale federal cutbacks of the first Reagan administration. Dr. Schwartz noticed something interesting, something he hadn't even been looking for. For whatever reason, children were going crazy in record numbers—or at least, so the printouts spread across his desk seemed to be saying.

Why were so many kids ending up in psychiatric hospitals? At first, Schwartz, a youth-policy expert with a growing national reputation, thought he was looking at a Minnesota phenomenon. The state had attracted more than its fair share of addiction messiahs and recovery proselytizers, who were drawn by Minnesota's alluring blend of affluence and political correctness. In the seventies, Minnesota was the first state to enact legislation requiring that employers provide mental-health benefits, including twenty-eight days of psychiatric inpatient treatment a year.

One result was certainly apparent in the Minneapolis–St. Paul area, where Schwartz found that the rate at which youths under eighteen were admitted to psychiatric units of general hospitals had doubled between 1977 and 1983. And that didn't even take into account the private psychiatric hospitals and substance-abuse centers that were just starting to open up shop. The Minnesota legislation mandating psychiatric inpatient coverage had "really opened up the barn door," Schwartz concluded.

Curious, Schwartz made some calls to colleagues in other states. Their checking supported what he had begun to suspect: All across the country, anecdotal information and sketchy statistical data suggested that kids were being channeled into psychiatric wards in unprecedented numbers.

Intrigued, Schwartz called Minnesota Blue Cross/Blue Shield. At first, Blue Cross couldn't say for sure. "They didn't really know—their records weren't broken down by age," Schwartz said. But then they did a more detailed computer search. "My God, you're right," a Blue Cross official told Schwartz.

The trend was even more pronounced in areas other than Minnesota, especially the Sunbelt.

"There was increased pressure by parents and others to do something for the out-of-control adolescent," explained Dr. Carl M. Pfeifer, a child psychiatrist who was chairman of the Texas Society of Psychiatric Physicians. "Some hospital administrators often made it easy for a patient to be admitted in this competitive atmosphere, and some psychiatrists, mostly unwittingly—occasionally wittingly—lost sight of their primary obligation to serve the patient and his family foremost. A treatment approach, psychiatric hospitalization, that was appropriate for a few began to be the answer for many. At times, greed seems to have become a stronger motive than service."

And, as Schwartz and others suspected, the hospitalization of adolescents had little to do with pressing medical needs. Rather, it was almost entirely "a market-driven phenomenon," said Mary Jane England, a child psychiatrist and former vice president for mental-health programs policy at Prudential Insurance. Since kids are easier to detain and more profitable to treat than adults, "we saw a mushrooming, 400 percent increase in adolescent beds across the country" in a few years' time. "In one year, a major chain of psychiatric hospitals spent $14 million on advertising. Their message was, if your child comes home from school with a D and runs to his room because he's upset, bring him down to our hospital for help. It was terrible. As long as they had insurance, they were admitted."

By 1989, children and adolescents accounted for well over $1 billion of the $3 billion paid to private psychiatric hospitals for inpatient treatment. Kids were staying in the hospital far longer— thirty-eight days on average, compared with twenty-two days for adults, according to statistics compiled by the National Association of Private Psychiatric Hospitals, the industry's main trade and lobby group. Kids also were charged far more; adolescents and children paid an average daily room-and-board rate of $510, compared with $432 for adults.

And the potential market for kids was growing, if one gave credence—as the news media routinely do—to pronouncements by federal mental-health experts. At the end of the 1980s, the National Institute of Mental Health—the federal government's chief agency for setting mental-health funding—declared as a matter of policy that *one fifth* of the more than 63 million U.S. children under the age of eighteen suffered from a diagnosable mental illness.

Dr. Breggin points to that as an example of the "half-cocked statistics" and "half-baked assertions" on which the psychiatric profession, closely aligned with federal health agencies and the hospital and pharmaceutical industries, tries to bolster what Professor Schwartz derides as "the myth that psychiatry is a science."

Still, scientific-sounding statistics such as the ones purporting to show that twenty percent of American kids are mentally ill are often accepted at face value by the press and on television, where "experts" have been telling the public for over a decade that a national mental-health crisis is raging.

In such an atmosphere, the psychiatric profession—which has had to contend with the low esteem of its medical peers ever since the days when psychiatrists functioned primarily as the custodians of insane asylums—began to see better times ahead for itself, now that so many Americans with long lives ahead of them, like children, were officially crazy. Behind the psychiatrists were aligned tens of thousands of nonphysicians—psychologists, counselors, and therapists—eager to enlist in the profitable battle to make America mentally "healthy."

In 1992, Richard Sarles, a past president of the American Society for Adolescent Psychiatry, which represents about five thousand child psychiatrists, assured *Psychiatric News*, the official organ of the American Psychiatric Association, that "approximately 20 percent of children and adolescents suffer from mental illnesses significant enough to require mental health services." He added, "As the field of adolescent psychiatry becomes more knowledgeable and sophisticated, we are identifying many children and adolescents who are manifesting severe psychopathology at younger and younger ages—most clinicians agree that children and adolescents are getting sicker younger."

Beyond that 20 percent of supposedly mentally ill kids are legions of adolescent rape and sexual-abuse victims, prostitutes, runaways, dropouts, unwed mothers, bulimics, alcohol, drug and nicotine addicts, even television and Nintendo addicts—all potential patients with a life of therapy (presumably paid for by private and/ or government insurance) ahead.

The psychiatric-hospital industry, of course, declares itself willing to do all it must in this time of crisis, if only government and insurers will heed the warnings and make more money available for treatment. Robert L. Trachtenberg, a former federal mental-health-policy official who left his government job to become executive director of the National Association of Private Psychiatric Hospitals, testified before Congress in 1992 that "on any given day . . . nearly eight million children suffer from mental illnesses." These kids are a vast "underserved population," he said, adding: "While eighty percent of children with physical handicaps receive services, less than thirty percent, and maybe less than twenty percent, of seriously emotionally disturbed children receive care."

What constitutes a serious emotional disturbance is, obviously, much harder to define—and much more open to questionable interpretation—than what constitutes a physical handicap. As policy researchers, such as Professor Schwartz, with no financial ties to the psychiatric industry were beginning to find, many of the kids ending up in the psychiatric ward were there not because they had a mental illness requiring hospitalization but because they had come into conflict with their parents. By the middle of the eighties, parental anxieties were being brilliantly exploited by aggressive marketing designed to sell psychiatric hospitalization as the answer to juvenile behavior problems and the key to household peace.

At the American Psychiatric Association's annual convention, opportunities in child psychiatry are avidly discussed. But ironically, the reputation of the founder of psychoanalysis, Sigmund Freud, has reached such a nadir among his biomedically oriented brethren that he is now respectfully cited usually only in justifying attention to childhood emotional trauma. Freud himself would not recognize the fast-paced modern world of biomedical psychiatry, with its emphasis on drugs, short-term "outcomes," and insurance reimbursement, and with its lack of interest in time-consuming talk or detailed analysis of an individual's complex emotions and personal experiences.

Still, federal mental-health studies assert that 50 percent of adults' mental disorders can be diagnosed in childhood. In the growth field of depression, new studies discussed at a recent APA convention purported to show that the number of *preschool-age* children already showing "clinically significant depression" is approaching 10 percent, with clear implications that a veritable epidemic of mental illness among teenagers could break out as these toddlers reach adolescence. Other studies, respectfully received, defined symptoms of depression and "low self-esteem" in infants, and sexual disorders in five-year-olds, as well as a "genetic marker" for criminal behavior in male black children.

This flood of revelation about endemic madness in the youth of America, and medicine's purported ability to confront it like a disease, like polio, caused one veteran psychiatrist, a psychoanalyst who prescribes drugs only as a last resort, to shake his head ruefully as he wandered among the forest of booths and displays promoting pharmaceutical companies and medical nostrums at the 1992 APA convention in Washington. "You think it's bad when the inmates are in charge of the asylum?" he asked. "It's worse when the shrinks are in charge."

Since emotional disorders first emerged as a political issue in the sixteenth century, the stresses of "modern times" have always been cited as a cause of mental illness.

By the 1980s, the American family was under mounting pressure as parents—both of whom, often, were employed—worked harder and longer just to stay even. A national survey found that the time American adults devoted to leisure activities fell from an average of 26.2 hours a week in 1973 to 16.6 hours a week in 1987. There was correspondingly less time to devote to both the joys and the travails of raising a child, especially a teenager.

At the same time, pharmaceutical companies were inventing new psychoactive drugs to treat children, and the psychiatric establishment was complying with business impulses to create new diagnoses designed specifically to meet insurance requirements for paying for the psychiatric hospitalization of increasing numbers of youths. Often, their targets were "basically just pain-in-the-ass kids, not psychotics, not insane," said Bill Johnson, the president of the National Association for Rights Protection and Advocacy in Minneapolis, a patients'-rights watchdog group. According to Peter Breggin: "In blaming the child-victim, psychiatry takes the pressure off the parents, the family, the schools, and the society."

Those new diagnoses were breathtaking in their scope. Consider the wide range of child and adolescent behaviors and classroom difficulties that are assigned official code numbers (keyed to insurance reimbursement) and classified as disorders in psychiatry's clinical bible, the *Diagnostic and Statistical Manual* (*DSM-III-R*).

Among them are numbers 315.10, "developmental arithmetic disorder," and 315.80, "developmental expressive writing disorder." One of the diagnoses most widely used to commit children and adolescents to a psychiatric hospital is number 313.81, "oppositional defiant disorder." In their entirety, here are the "diagnostic criteria" listed by *DSM-III-R*, a manifestation of only a few of which is sufficient to diagnose a child as mentally ill:

1. often loses temper
2. often argues with adults
3. often actively defies or refuses adult requests or rules, e.g., refuses to do chores at home
4. often deliberately does things that annoy other people, e.g., grabs other children's hats
5. often blames others for his or her mistakes
6. is often touchy or easily annoyed by others
7. is often angry and resentful
8. is often spiteful or vindictive
9. often swears or uses obscene language

As Professor Schwartz and others looking into the skyrocketing rates of psychiatric hospitalization of children have noted, it does not take a lot of effort to find a child to meet such criteria; at times such a child can be found in one's own home. The psychiatric industry created marketing plans with just that in mind.

When he began uncovering abuses and writing academic papers in the mid-80s, Schwartz didn't fully appreciate what he came to see as the ruthless nature of the business. "I was very naïve," he said. "When I found that intake workers at these hospitals were being paid bonuses for admitting kids, I said, Where I come from they call that taking kickbacks."

"I found these folks really stop at practically nothing to try to discredit somebody," he said. "A lot of the people in the hospital industry are evil. I'd really like to say they're not, but I've found it to be true. These are seedy people involved in a scam."

Schwartz later joined the faculty of the University of Michigan as the director of the Center for the Study of Youth Policy. In 1992, in his cluttered office in the center's headquarters in a rambling old house across the street from the campus in Ann Arbor, he recalled the thickets he had plowed through when he tried to understand why so many kids were being hospitalized.

"The first thing I was told was, Well, these kids all have serious mental-health problems. I looked at that. Not true. Then I was told, They all have serious problems with drugs or alcohol. That also wasn't true. Yes, there are some kids in these units with profound mental-health problems, with very serious problems with drugs or alcohol. But that's not the case with the overwhelming majority of them—and they all could be managed in a less intrusive environment."

Schwartz didn't expect to lead a crusade. "When I first got into this, studying the institutional problems, I was really kind of taken aback by it—the more I looked at it, the worse it looked." And the worse it got over the years, the more involved he became.

"I found primitive and abusive practices. Kids were being treated in such a way that if they were in a public facility, the facility would be under federal litigation for violating constitutional rights and for unconstitutional conditions of confinement. Kids are being abused. It's essentially child abuse and maltreatment."

One of Schwartz's major research projects showed the correlation between insurance coverage and length of stay in a psychiatric hospital. In 1991, he and a colleague, Jeffrey A. Butts, studied the records of 121,044 young people, aged thirteen to twenty-two, hospitalized for psychiatric treatment between 1986 and 1988. Eighty-two percent of the youths were white, and the group was about evenly split between males and females. Eighty percent were covered under private or government-funded insurance plans. The researchers showed conclusively that length of stay in the hospital was related to the amount of insurance that was available. At seven-day intervals, there were obvious peaks in discharges; this reflected insurance reimbursements typically paid in seven-day increments. Also, the younger a patient was, the longer he or she stayed in the hospital. And young patients were much more likely to have been hospitalized with a less serious diagnosis (one not involving psychosis), such as "adjustment reaction."

Professor Schwartz was blunt about the real nature of for-profit psychiatric hospitals. "Jails for middle-class kids," he called them.

Clinical interest in the mental health of children has some roots in nineteenth-century humanistic theories popularized early in this century by people like Dr. Maria Montessori, an Italian psychiatrist whose ideas about preschool learning environments greatly influenced the modern day-care center.

Long before the profit motive brought psychiatric bounty hunters to the schoolyard, psychiatrists envied the claim staked on the school-age market by psychologists and child-guidance counselors after the First World War, in an atmosphere of world publicity about the catastrophic social effects of war and epidemics on children and the family. By the 1950s, "child psychology" was a familiar term, conveying the now firmly established idea that psychoanalytic intervention, usually in a school or child-guidance clinic staffed by psychologists, was a way to protect the well-being of children.

In the fifties, public pressure to provide school services for physically handicapped children helped to establish a bureaucracy of special-education teachers, psychologists, and social workers. As years passed and that bureaucracy grew, its members became trained and authorized to intervene in matters affecting the emotional status of all children in the schools.

By the late sixties, federal health planners were seriously considering proposals to require that all children be given a baseline psychological screening at age two or three as a way to predict future problems. In the seventies, the impulse for intervention grew with the social backlash against the drug culture. In many schools, the tactics of private organizations, such as Synanon, that practiced confrontation were widely praised and imitated; concerns about coercion were generally discounted in the crusade against the evils of drugs. At the same time, billions of federal dollars revolutionized the hospital business, creating a thriving industry based on making as much money as possible. When that industry in turn discovered the profits available in psychiatry, it was only natural that the schools would become centers of intense interest.

At the same time, the American family was undergoing a transition on a scale not seen since the industrial revolution. Adrift in a transient and rootless society, buffeted by divorce, reshaped by the fact that both father and mother now usually were employed outside the home, confused and frightened by incessant alarms about teenagers' rampant drug addiction, alienation, and suicide, the American family of the Reagan era was a prime marketing opportunity, and the rapidly expanding psychiatric-hospital industry, voraciously hungry, saw a big payoff in kids.

In an increasingly medicalized society, the payoff was huge for psychiatric hospitals claiming to offer cures that were not only convenient and effective, but also could be had without financial pain, since insurance—as the advertising always pointed out—paid the bill.

Critics of the psychiatric-hospital industry don't dispute the assertion that a certain percentage of the nation's children and adolescents need mental-health treatment, some of them critically. But very few of them need to be hospitalized to get it. However, government policies and insurance reimbursement practices all are keyed to inpatient treatment amid, Schwartz said, "intense competition to capture a share of the market and turn a profit."

As the psychiatric industry swept up large groups of children, even states with a tradition of closely regulating hospitals found themselves overwhelmed. In 1990, a report was commissioned by the Illinois legislature in defense of state legislation regulating hospital growth against fierce lobbying by private psychiatric hospitals. The report stated that the number of psychiatric beds for minors had already increased 66 percent in Illinois between 1985 and 1988. State health authorities attributed the trend to the link between for-profit hospitals and insurance benefits favoring inpatient treatment. Warning of the "dramatic" increase in psychiatric hospitalization of "a select group of adolescents"—those whose parents had liberal insurance coverage—the report noted that many kids who actually seemed to need treatment, but didn't have insurance, were being "processed" in another way: by the criminal justice system.

But the psychiatric establishment largely ignored the growing problem, despite an article in *Psychiatric Times* in 1987 entitled "Psychiatry's Time Bomb." The author, Adam Blatner, warned that the "proliferation of private psychiatric hospitals . . . poses a major threat to the psychiatric profession. It generates a significant pressure for admitting patients and keeping them in the hospital. . . . It is only a matter of time until the public, consumer groups, and [insurers] become aware of this situation."

Here and there outside academia, other small warnings were being heard.

In Los Angeles County, a mental-health official warned in a memo on "teenaged mental patients" being placed in private hospitals in 1983: "These facilities really are being used as detention centers and reform schools, not as hospitals." The official, Ralph Lopez, chief of the Health Facilities Division of the Los Angeles County Department of Health Services, cautioned county officials in charge of certifying hospitals that the private psychiatric facilities then opening all over California were "preying on parents' fears."

Lopez concluded: "These issues need to be faced and resolved before the lid blows off somewhere."

CHAPTER SIX

....

FEW OF THE KIDS VICTIMIZED BY PSYCHIATRIC HOSPITALS ARE carted off against their parents' wishes the way Jeramy Harrell was in San Antonio. The vast majority are sent away by their parents. With rising alarm in the 1980s about drugs and alcohol, teenage pregnancy and suicide, and other troubles, anxious parents and schools were receptive to new approaches. Given the time constraints of modern parenting, solutions that could be purchased like tennis lessons or orthodontic braces were attractive, especially when the adults were assured that everything would be taken care of in one neat package—even the cost, thanks to insurance.

Skillful marketing strategies were devised, appealing to insecurity and opportunity and offering to take pressure off parents and schools. The ads are "very seductive and misleading," said Ira Schwartz. "They essentially tell parents this message: 'If your child is having difficulty, you owe it to yourself, as a responsible parent, to bring your child into our hospital for diagnostic assessment.' If you don't, the ads usually say, something very terrible can happen to your child. They could end up in jail, or committing suicide. In addition, of course, the ads remind parents that their insurance will pick up the tab." Often, such advertising "stressed the tragedy of suicide and warned parents that *their* teenager might be a prime candidate for self-violence if he seemed sulky," added Frank P. Schuster, a psychiatrist who had noticed the phenomenon.

"A lot of these kids and their parents are at war with each other," Schwartz said. "It's a hell of a lot easier for a parent to be told: 'Look, this isn't your problem. Johnny is depressed and rebellious because it's really a mental-health problem. It's not your problem, and we know how to fix it. Send Johnny to us.' "

The calculated appeal is that "it absolves a parent of guilt because they can say, 'I'm not part of that problem, and I don't even have to be part of the solution—there's just something wrong with Johnny. Johnny will go away—not to jail, but to the people in the white coats, all sanitized and palatable, and he'll come home fixed.' "

Instead, "Johnny comes home bitter and angry about being hospitalized unnecessarily. It becomes really sort of a nasty game. Very few of these programs provide any real family-oriented services—the problems really don't go away. They get exacerbated.

"These places are pretty primitive; the quality of treatment is not very good. They're actually amazing—the behavior-modification regimes and token economies they use are right out of the training schools of the fifties and sixties that we got rid of: youth correctional facilities, reform schools. These psychiatric hospitals and mental-health units are the new training schools. We have had a long-standing love affair with locking up kids and trying to control kids with detention. As a society, we have always incarcerated kids."

Obviously, the advertising has been working. To a degree that professional child counselors from other countries find astonishing, some American mothers and fathers commit their children to psychiatric hospitals as casually as they would send them to summer camp. And by the end of the decade, with the costs of psychiatric hospitalization rising twice as fast as medical costs generally, the cost of psychiatric hospitalization of children and adolescents was going up even faster. Analysts estimate it was rising at 300 to 350 percent a year by the end of the decade.

The for-profit psychiatric hospitalization of adolescents and children reached a frenzy at the end of the 1980s. But dire warnings about growing abuses in this area were being issued as early as 1980, well before the worst violations occurred.

In 1984, the Rand Corporation, a California think tank, expressed serious reservations about questionable claims being made by psychiatric hospitals for treating children. Rand analysts pointed out that no reliable data existed to indicate that in-hospital treatment was any better than outpatient treatment in the majority of cases. A Rand study of methods for controlling adolescent drug abuse found no value in building more inpatient facilities and cautioned that "a major expansion of treatment resources for adolescents would lack a sound basis."

But a major expansion is exactly what occurred.

Community Psychiatric Centers (CPC), like its competitors in the industry, embarked on a big construction drive at just that time. In 1986, CPC opened seven new psychiatric hospitals. The next year, it opened seven more, and four more in each of the two succeeding years. In CPC's 1988 annual report, the company chairman, Robert L. Green, and its president, James W. Conte, wrote a letter to stockholders that boasted of the aggressive search for new patients in places such as schools:

"A top priority for the company is the continuing development of new programs . . ." they wrote. "In 1988, significant gains have been achieved and are primarily attributable to growing community awareness of our programs for treatment of children, alcohol and drug abuse, sexual abuse, eating disorders. . . . The company's community education and marketing programs . . . have become more extensive and effective."

The executives proudly reported that "over 60 percent of referrals to our hospitals now originate in the community without the initial involvement of a psychiatrist. These referrals are received, often as the result of [community] outreach programs, from the clergy, school counselors, and teachers, the judicial and law enforcement system, employee assistance programs maintained by many corporations, and from the emergency rooms of many hospitals."

Psychiatric hospitals like to claim that most of their patients come in by referral from physicians. But the trend in recent years has been different: Most patients are coming in as a direct result of advertising and promotion, which leads them to a company-employed psychiatrist, who signs the papers for admission.

Political pressure from the industry eased the way for psychiatric hospitals to expand even in states where regulatory officials tried to resist. In 1986, Tennessee hospital regulators received thirteen applications for new or expanded psychiatric facilities for children, said Professor Schwartz; the corporations applying mounted "intensive lobbying campaigns" to get approval, even though the commissioner of the state Mental Health and Retardation Department had said that Tennessee was already "seriously overbedded with child and adolescent psychiatric beds."

In Arkansas, nine new private psychiatric hospitals with children's and adolescent wings opened between 1985 and 1990. Another one, Pinnacle Pointe Hospital, was opened by CPC the following next year in Little Rock. Marilyn Means, a director of clinical services at the hospital, described the typical young patients as "kids that parents don't want at birthday parties—the ones that are tough to control."

But unpopular kids were only part of the market targeted by massive campaigns of marketing and advertising to fill those new beds. While advertising evokes anxieties caused by rootless families, two-career parents, alienation, rebellion, drugs, and sex, there is often a subtle suggestion that psychiatric hospitalization of a child can also provide long-suffering parents with an all-expense-paid respite from their troublesome children.

"Many parents see this type of program as a way to get a rest from the ill-behaved child at someone else's expense," said Walter Afield, a Florida psychiatrist who founded a consulting firm that reviews mental-health treatment for employers worried about insurance costs.

Any parent of a teenager, and most adults who remember being teenagers, knows that it isn't difficult to detect irrational behavior at certain points in puberty or adolescence. "Most kids look psychotic at various times in their lives," Afield pointed out. When psychiatric-hospital administrators are eager to fill beds, "these kids can be admitted and kept for a long period of time," Afield said. However, there are consequences that the reassuring advertising never mentions. Psychiatric hospitalization "labels them with a diagnosis forever" on their medical records, Afield noted, with potential future problems in employment and in obtaining health-insurance coverage.

Russell D. Durrett, who was the chief controller at an NME psychiatric hospital in Denton, Texas, until he was dismissed for challenging its policies in 1989, said that many of the kids he encountered had friends or classmates who had also been incarcerated by their parents and were making the best of it. "Their attitude was, This is the in-thing to do, spend the summer in a psychiatric hospital," he said.

Psychiatric marketing for children often pays close attention to seasonal opportunities to exploit familial stress. One popular strategy is to intensify advertising during the occasions when parents are most focused on their children's performance—for example, report-card and exam times.

In 1988, Charter Palms Hospital, a Charter Medical psychiatric institution in McAllen, Texas, distributed a memo to its employees encouraging them to recruit for a program designed for adolescents with attitude problems. It said in part:

> *The customers are parents of underachieving students. Parents become most concerned during the school year when report cards arrive. Heavy marketing should coincide with the arrival of the report cards.*

In Reno, Nevada, an HCA-owned private psychiatric institution, Truckee Meadows Hospital, ran ads in the spring of 1991 depicting a report card with D's and F's, and a teacher's scrawled note to a parent: "Please see me about Rickey's grades." The ad warns: "The child who brought this home may have Attention Deficit Disorder. We can help."

HCA hospitals in Nevada ran such advertisements for over three years in the state's three biggest newspapers on the days that report cards in the state's largest school districts were issued. According to Curtis Decker, director of the patients'-rights group, "many parents who took their children in for an evaluation in response to the advertisement were told by the staff that it would be necessary to admit the children for evaluation and treatment. Many parents admitted their child and a long course of treatment followed . . . terminated only when their benefits ran out." Decker's organization dispatched an investigating team, which found that once admitted, some children were disciplined by "extended periods of detention (up to 13 hours a day for up to seven consecutive months)," and others "were forced to stand holding their ankles for up to 90 minutes at a time."

Charter Pacific Hospital, near Los Angeles, ran ads that said: "Is your teen failing life? Another school year is ending, and your teenager is farther behind . . . oppositional . . . becoming more difficult . . . constantly pushing the limits. You feel that you are losing control. You're scared to death that drugs are involved." With vacation season coming, the solution to having such a problem around the house was obvious: "This summer is the time to inter-vene in a more drastic fashion," the ad urges. "Call and ask for the admission coordinator."

(Charter Medical, long admired in the industry for having the most aggressive and most compelling advertising, claimed to take its mission seriously. In the company's 1986 annual report, Chart-er's founder and president, William A. Fickling, Jr., described the marketing as representing "a moral obligation to tell those who need our help that we understand their problem and that we offer quality services that can help make them a better person.")

Some of the most impressive and ambitious marketing involved contracting with shuttle services to arrange door-to-door pickup and delivery of youthful psychiatric patients.

In California, the benign-sounding "Teen Hospital Shuttle" began riding the San Fernando Valley in the middle of the 1980s, dropping in unexpectedly on some youths at home, and sometimes taking them away in restraints to private psychiatric hospitals, usu-ally at the behest of a parent unwilling to confront the child directly.

The Teen Shuttle advertised itself as a service for "the caring and safe transportation" of troubled adolescent children. With a hospital admission order, Teen Shuttle would notify law enforce-ment agencies first and then dispatch "a team. This unique working relationship with law enforcement agencies throughout Southern California enhances Teen Shuttle's ability to handle any situation."

Parents were assured that Teen Shuttle employees identified themselves properly and explained that they were there to help influence a child "to abide by their parents' desires to see them receive treatment. Their health and well-being are first and foremost."

Decker's organization gathered affidavits from youths and parents affirming that children were "physically assaulted, handcuffed, dragged out of their homes." And many of the kids came home under the influence of one psychotropic drug or another. "We were told that in order to make sure you can receive reimbursement from insurance companies you have to medicate the child, because if the child is not receiving medication that possibly represents a red flag to the insurance companies that maybe the child isn't sick enough to really be in the facility," Decker said.

In Los Angeles County and neighboring Orange County, a similar service was called Teen Rescue. Its ads promised:

> *Teen Rescue will locate your runaway teenager, safely transport them to a Teen Rescue care unit, and provide them with counseling services and free drug testing. If your child is out of control, involved in criminal behavior, abusing or using drugs or alcohol or has run away from home, call us for a free evaluation or consultation.*

Almost invariably, investigators found that free consultation began with questions about the extent of the parents' insurance coverage.

The promotional material made no mention of the psychiatric hospital where many of the kids ended up once their insurance was verified. "What the teenager needs is an in-between stage, a place where they can feel safe, comfortable, and reestablish communication and hopefully trust and respect with their parents. . . . Teen Rescue will actually go out and find the runaway if necessary. However, instead of taking them home, troubled teens are transported directly to the Alpha Teen Care Unit where professional Christian counselors have time to evaluate the emotional, physical and relational treatments needed to help each runaway eventually return home. . . . Your prayers for the absent child have not gone unanswered."

These ads "prey on the parents' uncertainty and apparent lack of options," Decker said. On the other hand, for many kids who actually need help, competent crisis counseling and treatment are out of reach because there isn't a profit in them. "Many of these kids could be helped at a community-based mental-health outpatient center. But they either are not available, or the parents do not know they exist."

While four big national corporations account for seven out of ten for-profit psychiatric beds in the United States, dozens of other chain operators and single-facility institutions are in the business, and many are just as innovative in their marketing and advertising as the corporate giants. Here are some examples from all sectors of the business:

• "Suicide Among Youth in Virginia," warns one newsletter from a chain of for-profit crisis centers associated with Tidewater Psychiatric Institute, an NME hospital in Norfolk. "The national suicide rate has tripled since 1950. . . . There are an estimated 500 to 1,000 suicide attempts by adolescents for each completed suicide. . . . The number of suicides might be higher, because deaths among children under 10 that might be suicides are officially listed as accidents."

• "Attitudes in Teenage Addiction: Sex, Satan & Suicide," blares the type atop an ad for Charter Hospital of Las Vegas, announcing a free program in which "nationally acclaimed" child psychiatrist Paul King, M.D., will lecture on "the relationship between Heavy Metal Music, Drugs, Sex, Satan & Suicide."

• During the Persian Gulf war, Tidewater Psychiatric Institute in Virginia Beach, Virginia, an area where several large military installations are located, advertised a "support group" program for parents of military personnel serving in Desert Storm.

• A magazine ad for Charter Pacific Hospital, near Los Angeles, deftly combines anxiety about anger toward a child with an assurance of help, impeccably underlaid by irreproachable concern about the problem of child abuse. The ad features a cartoon with an exasperated mother in an apron shaking her fist at her wailing toddler. "He's *never* gonna outgrow it!" the cartoon mother cries. The copy advises, "Don't hit him. Call now, day or night."

• College Hospital, "A Psychiatric Center for Behavioral Medicine" in Cerritos, California, ran ads showing distraught parents outside a jail cell where their son is behind bars. "What went wrong?" the ad asks. Whatever did, it is most likely a medical matter, not a social one, the ad strongly suggests: "Studies indicate that anti-social behaviors in adolescents usually are not 'reactions' to home, school or community involvements. They, more often than not, are disorders of *neurological development.*"

• Charter Hospital of Long Beach, California, listed a twenty-four-hour "crisis line" with this appeal to worried parents: "Our staff works with parents of teens to recognize emotional and behavioral problems such as withdrawal and depression, acts of defiance and rebellion and drug or alcohol abuse [which indicate] inner conflict. . . . We put teenagers back on course."

• St. Francis Academy Inc., with a number of hospitals in Kansas and New York, ran ads warning ominously of "conduct disorders" in children who "find it difficult to function in their environments." The answer? Hospitalization—or, as the ad put it, "a 24-hour structured milieu [that] emphasizes a holistic approach" to psychiatric confinement. "We are CHAMPUS and insurance-certified," the ad notes.

All across the country, psychiatric hospitals present parents with frightening illustrations of their worst fears concerning their teenagers. Ads run nationally by the Children's Division of the Menninger Foundation in Topeka, Kansas, pictured a despondent boy behind a door with a hand-lettered sign reading "Jason's Room. KEEP OUT!" Parents are cautioned that many adolescent problems "do not respond to outpatient or brief inpatient treatment." Charter

Pacific Hospital in Torrance, California, showed a boy with his hands cuffed behind his back and the word "BUSTED" spelled out boldly above his head. "Don't wait until you get a call from the police to get help for your teenager," the ad warns. In Virginia, ads for Psychiatric Institute of Richmond, an NME hospital, state: "If a child is changing before your eyes, we have special care for special kids." Ads for Camelback Hospitals in Scottsdale, Arizona, show the face of a troubled boy above the message "He Shouldn't Be Living at Home Right Now." The message also subtly criticizes outpatient treatment and short-stay hospitalization: "Rebuilding takes time," it says.

Scare tactics are obviously effective. In 1992, *Hospital and Community Psychiatry* published the results of a survey designed to gauge the impact of psychiatric hospitals' "fear-based advertising." The subjects of the survey were a group of mothers of high school students. Overwhelmingly, the women were well-educated and middle-class, and lived in two-parent households. The group was asked to rate, for "fear arousal," twelve different newspaper ads from psychiatric hospitals looking for adolescent patients. When the women were next asked which ads were most likely to cause them to seek services, the most frightening ones scored highest. But the intriguing implication found by the study was that scare ads worked best on the people whose children were least troubled. The study's authors, Sue Greer and Paul Greenbaum, concluded that "frightening advertising for psychiatric hospitals arouses more fear among those who least need mental health services and less fear among those for whom the services may be more useful."

But the marketing isn't all doom and gloom; indeed, much of it tends to be sunny and reassuring, with positive illustrations of joyful results, such as an ad that shows a happy, tousled-haired boy of about nine displaying a mathematics test with an A+ scrawled on top. "Made Possible by Charter Hospital of San Diego," it says. "We teach your child to be the best he can be!"

Another favorite strategy is to introduce psychiatric hospitalization with solicitations to what sound like family outings. In their zeal to fill beds, psychiatric hospitals routinely troll for toddlers with promotions for on-grounds fairs and child-oriented events like puppet shows, designed to lure parents to bring their children in for "evaluation." Charter Hospital in Sioux Falls, South Dakota, offered free teddy bears to children who came by with parents for special events. Charter hospitals in the Los Angeles area sponsored "Youth at Risk Fairs," five-hour events with refreshments, gifts, and entertainment on the hospital grounds, "offering your son or daughter the opportunity to get a mental health check-up." Some of these programs offered assessments of emotional outlook, chemical-dependence indicators, family and school problems, nutrition concerns, and one ad even promised a "spiritual needs assessment."

Others implore apprehensive parents to be aware of dark signs of trouble. "Kathy's parents are successful professionals," says an ad for Meridell Achievement Center, a long-term psychiatric hospital in Austin, Texas. "They are confused and frustrated with the stranger their daughter has become during her teen years. Kathy has become moody and angry at home." Another Meridell ad, depicting a high-school girl with downcast eyes, is headlined "Adolescent Depression: The Silent Enemy" and stresses the benefits of long-term hospitalization: "After being in a short-term psychiatric hospital, Cindi is still depressed and has made suicidal gestures."

A series of ads by Del Amo Hospital, a facility near Los Angeles owned by the big hospital chain American Medical International, shows head shots of brooding youngsters aged five to seventeen, and lists under each one symptoms of disorders including "unable to function in school," "developmental impairment," and "suicidal." Another Del Amo ad shows a sullen young boy with the warning "Sometimes It's Not Just a Phase . . ."

Professor Schwartz and others appalled by the wanton psychiatric hospitalization of young people use the term "medicalization of

defiance" to describe the tactic of luring parents into sending kids
to a mental hospital for behavior that would have merely gotten
them sent to the woodshed in years past. Among the favored diagnoses psychiatrists affiliated with these institutions employ to
hospitalize such children are "oppositional defiant disorder" and
the all-encompassing "conduct disorder" and "adolescent adjustment disorder." By 1990, these three diagnoses accounted for over
a third of all psychiatric admissions for adolescents and children.

In Kentucky in 1990, investigators for a national patients'-rights
organization found that 80 percent of the kids at one private psychiatric hospital were there with a diagnosis of "conduct disorder."

"Oppositional" and "defiant" behaviors are buzzwords in adolescent hospitalization. Ads run by NME's Alvarado Parkway Institute in San Diego depict a child with his hands on hips and warn
ominously of "Defiant behavior, such as refusing to obey, clean
rooms or shower . . ." Sometimes the defiance is subtle: "Is Your
Teenager Running Away Without Leaving Home?" asks an ad run
by Comprehensive Care Corporation's adolescent hospitals in the
Los Angeles area.

Sometimes the diagnoses themselves are self-perpetuating.

"In the hospital setting, the newly admitted adolescent is particularly likely to be oppositional, defensive and resistant," David
Greenfield, a clinical professor of psychiatry at Yale University
School of Medicine, wrote in *Psychiatric Annals* in 1992. "Once
in the hospital, adolescents . . . may feel obliged to remain because
their parents refuse to allow them to return home. The resulting
resentment can be reflected in opposition to clinicians whom they
see as agents of their parents."

Ira Schwartz cited an Illinois study showing that in 1986, before the heaviest marketing got under way, two thirds of youths
discharged from hospitals with psychiatric problems had nonpsycho-
tic diagnoses, and 80 percent of *those* were adjustment or conduct disorders. As for those who *were* diagnosed as psychotic, a
significant portion had experienced only one episode of major

depression. Of those hospitalized for drug or alcohol use, half were classified "nondependent."

Advertising and promotion are the most publicly visible layers of hospitals' meticulously crafted strategies to keep beds filled, at almost any cost. Within hospital marketing departments, where the need to fill beds and keep referrals active was constantly stressed, disgruntled and overworked staff employees grumbled that terms such as "product line" and "buyer behavior" were constantly heard, but that "patient care" was not. One said: "It was like I was working for Amway, not for a hospital."

In 1989, Charter Brook Hospital in Atlanta issued to employees a memo describing a "90-day marketing plan" to "reposition" the hospital "as the *only* alternative for adolescent chemical dependency treatment." The memo spoke of "sales expectations" and specified monthly "census goals" for admitting more adolescents.

In businesslike detail the memo spelled out the hospital's objectives for improving relationships with "referral markets"—teachers, coaches, school administrators, and other professionals in regular contact with young people. The hospital's "Spiritual Counselor" was recommended as a liaison to develop contacts with clergy members in the area, and training area teachers was cited as a means to identify "high-risk" students. The memo pointed out the opportunities for developing referrals from lawyers who handle juvenile cases. It advised: "Target juvenile probation officers."

The memo also recommended strategies for enhancing the institution's reputation with the local news media, suggesting that employees speak of it "as a facility you can 'trust' " and even pointing out that Charter Brook Hospital's name itself offered opportunites for image enhancement: "Emphasize 'BROOK.' "

Image enhancement remains paramount. In 1993, ads for a seventy-two-bed psychiatric hospital named National Hospital for Kids in Crisis ("Ending their Pain") listed its address as KidsPeace Drive

in Orefield, Pennsylvania. The toll-free phone number: 1-800-44-
MY-KID.

Curtis Decker shook his head ruefully as he inspected the ad showing the beaming youngster of about nine and captioned: "Made
Possible by Charter Pacific Hospital." Decker said he wasn't quite
sure that it was meant to convey to distraught parents facing a
crisis, except, perhaps: "if you send your child in here, he'll come
back out blond and smiling and bright, I guess."

A child never forgets the experience of being sent to a psychiatric
hospital. "When you look at the process of how these children
make it into these facilities, you can see abuses at every step in
the process," Decker said. Marketing is the most obvious one.
There are more personal ones, however, such as the sense of be-
trayal left in the mind of a youngster who has been sent to a
psychiatric ward by his or her parents, and the ill effects on the
family, which can persist for years.

"We have reports of many children refusing to return home
because they feel betrayed by their parents, even though the parents may have had good intentions in trying to seek treatment for
their child," Decker said. "So not only does the child receive a
great deal of damage in the course of their treatment, but it lives
long after their experience in the psychiatric facility."

The strain on family trust isn't the only time bomb ticking in
teenagers who feel they have been unjustly confined to a psychiatric
hospital. There also is a legacy of cynicism, with long-term implications for the social and political attitudes of the first generation
of Americans for whom psychiatric hospitalization is a familiar
event, if not for themselves then for someone they have known or
heard about personally.

"Youths here in Reno who enter the hospital under the impression that they are there for a 'ten-day evaluation' soon learn from
their peers that they will remain in the hospital for as long as they

have insurance coverage," recalled Dr. Kenneth M. Clark, a Nevada psychiatrist who told congressional investigators about abuses in a Hospital Corporation of America facility there where he was on the staff. Few teenagers are fooled by the advertising, which they consider to be just another hustle in a consumer economy where anything can be sold. At corporate-owned psychiatric hospitals, young patients openly joke about the correlation between insurance coverage and length of stay. Dr. Clark spoke of a Seattle girl whose parents were divorcing and who "had the misfortune of having a one-million-dollar John Hancock insurance policy" for psychiatric hospitalization. After weeks of frustration, the girl's mother finally hired a prominent Seattle psychiatrist who managed to get the teenager released only after filing a petition with Nevada juvenile authorities. The psychiatrist questioned why that hospital in Reno had two and a half times as many adolescent patients as all of the hospitals in Seattle combined, Dr. Clark said.

Nevada has less stringent legal protection for teenagers who claim abuse by a psychiatric hospital than other states in the region. Seattle-area insurance carriers, alarmed about abuses, had sharply cut back on psychiatric-reimbursement levels for children and adolescents. In California, furthermore, a minor over fourteen who demands a hearing to protest psychiatric confinement is entitled to one. Clark estimated that as a result, about one third of the adolescent patients in his Reno hospital at any time were from California.

Some of the worst examples of cynical marketing surfaced in Texas, where school districts unwittingly employed counselors who were secretly linked to the marketing operations of private psychiatric hospitals, which in turn provided money to set up "student assistance programs" that were little more than means to identify potential new customers, much as a traditional sales force uses referrals and other information to identify leads.

In some districts, the "student assistance programs" involved the distribution of evaluation forms for use by high school and junior high school students and faculty to facilitate tips on referrals. "Intervention specialists"—actually, marketing employees from private psychiatric hospitals—were provided to advise counselors on treatment for identified students. The programs established in schools revolved around "Core Teams," small groups of teachers and counselors, who met "at least twice a month" to evaluate student referral forms and "make appropriate referrals to community resources."

The "referral" tips, contained on four-page "Behavior of Concern" forms, were informal, to say the least—considering that anyone could use them. "Anyone can submit a 'Behavior of Concern' referral for a student: teachers, counselors, nurses, aides, custodians, concerned community members, parents and students themselves," material for one such program proclaimed. Completed forms were submitted anonymously to "student assistance counselors," school employees who could—and did—receive secret payments from psychiatric hospitals for each kid they referred for "evaluation" by hospital personnel.

When this program became known in some school districts in Texas, one parent's first reaction was to think of her own high school years. "It was just the kind of thing you would need to make life miserable for your biggest enemy on the prom committee," she said with an uneasy laugh, after she had read the blank "Behavior of Concern" form her ninth-grade daughter brought home from school:

> If you or another student exhibit(s) several of the following behaviors of concern, it probably indicates the need for referral to the Student Assistance Program. In order for the team to have reliable information to base our review on, it is necessary for the person referring a student to report actual OBSERVABLE information.
>
> Directions: please answer questions about behaviors either you or another student have *experienced or observed.* Check

the frequency in the response column. Additional comments would be helpful and can be written on the back of the form. Return the form to your counselor or a teacher in an envelope marked "confidential."

ACADEMIC

Has he/she

_____ Had a drop in grades or failing grades?

_____ Been caught or told you about cheating?

_____ Refused/protested changing clothes for Physical Education?

ATTENDANCE

Has he/she

_____ Been tardy in the last six weeks?

_____ Been absent in the last six weeks?

_____ Skipped school during the last six weeks?

PHYSICAL SYMPTOMS

Has he/she

_____ Slept in class?

_____ Gained or lost weight in the last six months?

_____ Felt fatigued or drowsy during school?

_____ Experienced slurred speech?

_____ Experienced increasing nervousness or paranoia?

_____ Had runny nose or respiratory illness in the last six weeks?

_____ Had an injury they tried to hide or not talk about?

_____ Had skin marks they tried to hide or lie about?

_____ Visited the nurse frequently?

ALCOHOL/DRUGS

Does he/she

_____ Have drugs or drug paraphernalia in possession?

_____ Talk openly about using alcohol (beer) or drugs?

_____ Get involved with illegal activities?

_____ Read drug-related magazines?

_____ Use liquor in addition to beer?

_____ Use other drugs in addition to pot?

_____ Been afraid to run out of beer, pot or other drugs?

PEERS

Does he/she

_____ Have (new) friends involved in drinking or drugs?

_____ Exclude "straights" from activities?

_____ Engage in drinking contests (drinks more than should)?

_____ Withdrawn from friends? Been a loner?

_____ Felt others don't care about likes/dislikes?

_____ Gone beyond acceptable limits/their conscience in sexual behavior?

SOCIAL PROBLEMS

Has he/she

_____ Had problems with a boss/coworker on a job?

_____ Visited a school counselor in the past six weeks?

_____ Failed to keep commitments with teachers, counselors, coaches, family?

_____ Had a death, divorce or serious illness in the family?

DISRUPTIVE BEHAVIOR

Does he/she

_____ Laugh/show anger at inappropriate times?

_____ Use language offensive to adults?

_____ Argue with teachers, family, friends?

_____ Feel/show hostility/anger/dislike toward others?

_____ Make threatening statements?

_____ Blame others? Deny own behavior?

_____ Get sent to detention?

ATYPICAL BEHAVIOR

Has he/she

_____ Been depressed in the last six weeks?

_____ Had mood swings: Real happy one day, sad/de-pressed/worried the next?

_____ Lied to teachers or parents about activities/friends?

_____ Attempted suicide?

Said the astonished mother of one Texas teenager: "Every kid I have ever known qualifies for a referral!"

CHAPTER SEVEN

....

FEW PATIENTS, CHILDREN OR ADULTS, ARE ADMITTED TO A psychiatric hospital without the assent of a psychiatrist. And few of the many thousands of American psychiatrists who are affiliated with for-profit psychiatric hospitals raised public objections to the high-pressure tactics used throughout the industry to keep beds full. Some finally had enough and blew the whistle, however.

Among them was a California psychiatrist named Corydon G. Clark. In 1992, Dr. Clark came forward with this admission about his own role in hospitalizing kids:

"I have personally participated in every aspect of the unscrupulous and deceptive practices. I can state with complete confidence that at least 65 percent of all these admissions were not medically necessary. Distressed families are, in my opinion, routinely presented (by admissions staffs) a very misleading portrayal of services and benefits their child would receive during hospitalization. Psychiatrists, during the evaluation process that follows admission, routinely commit what amounts to fraud by concocting diagnoses which are more in tune with what they know the insurance will reimburse than actual psychiatric disorder evident. . . . Thousands of children and adolescents and their parents are directly harmed every day by the current system."

125

Norton A. Roitman, an adolescent psychiatrist, said he was recruited in 1988 to head the adolescent unit of a private psychiatric
hospital in las Vegas. Once on board, he was amazed to find a
hospital staff utterly "ignorant of basic psychiatric principles." But
the main reason he quit within a year was this: "The incentive in
that system would most likely have led me to compromise my
values." Roitman tabulated an amazing array of opportunities for
profiteering for unscrupulous physicians, including the ability to
bill $80 to $125 a day for spending a "minimal" amount of time
with a patient. There was no barrier, he said, to billing $2,500 a
day, seven days a week, doing little more than attending a few
meetings and "making sure my charts were neat." Roitman was
especially troubled by the hospital's insistence that, in their initial
phase of hospitalization, teenagers be kept from seeing their parents. This was presented as a way to encourage "bonding" to the
hospital. "It was general knowledge," he recalled, "that the purpose
of it was so that the adolescent patient would not talk the parents
out of the forced hospitalization."

Hal Chandler, a psychiatrist in Oklahoma City, worked in PIA
psychiatric hospitals for three years, and said he was increasingly
"concerned that the administration placed too much emphasis on
making a profit and too little emphasis on the actual well-being of
patients." Among other abuses, he noticed, patients were kept in
the hospital unnecessarily, "until insurance benefits were exhausted," and there was inadequate follow-up care. The hospitals
were interested chiefly in "looking for immediate profit," Chandler
said, adding that there were clear rewards for going along since
affiliated psychiatrists were assigned patients on the basis of their
"length of stay" records.

Until the 1980s, most psychological work with children involved
counseling and therapy, more often conducted by a psychologist
or a trained social worker than by a psychiatrist. But even when a
psychiatrist was involved, therapy was usually in the form of talk.

The rise of medically oriented "biopsychiatrists," who now dominate psychiatry, accompanied the rapid growth in for-profit mental hospitals and the sharp increases in the number of children confined in psychiatric hospitals since 1980. In the decade since that trend intensified, a new specialty has gained prominence: "pediatric pharmacotherapy." This involves treating young children with antidepressants and other mood-altering drugs to correct malfunctions in the metabolism of brain neurotransmitters. Psychiatrists claim that chemical short circuits can cause certain behavior problems in children, notably hyperactivity, and can indicate a potential for later drug and alcohol abuse.

Hyperactivity as a medical diagnosis increased abruptly in the 1980s. In one study of American teachers (cited in a 1981 book, *Hyperactive Children: A Handbook for Diagnosis and Treatment*, by psychologist Russell Barkley) 57 percent of the boys and 42 percent of the girls in American public schools were labeled hyperactive. In his 1991 book *Toxic Psychiatry*, psychiatrist Peter Breggin cites a 1989 *Clinical Psychiatry News* report of a Duke University study demonstrating that "the amount of trouble that children are causing adults, particularly teachers, appears to be the driving force determining children's referrals to mental health services."

Some authorities scoffed at the notion that vaguely defined maladies with precise-sounding names like child "attention deficit disorder" affected such a large population of kids. Nevertheless, the psychiatric establishment worked assiduously to provide clinical validity for treating such problems as medical illnesses. By 1987, *DSM-III-R* listed attention deficit disorder with hyperactivity as a specific mental illness. According to one critic, "most of the routine problems of growth and development" now met criteria to be classified as mental disorders. Meanwhile, Breggin carefully went through the *DSM-III-R* and added up the top estimated incidence of each "school-related" disorder. According to the manual's statistics, 60 percent of *all American children* would be suffering from one or another mental disorder, he calculated.

Yet despite all the scientific-sounding diagnoses and pronounce-ments, the reality of psychiatric hospitals for children, besides med-ication, is a quotidian routine often enforced with disciplinary techniques that have been discredited since the days of the "snake pit" asylums.

"One of the most alarming issues surrounding the hospitaliza-tions of children and youths for psychiatric and substance abuse is the fact that some of the programs are abusive and degrading," Schwartz wrote in the *Journal of Adolescent Health Care* in 1989.

> *They typically consist of rigid and punitive "behavior modifi-cation" regimes . . . characterized by excessive and sometimes lengthy use of isolation and solitary confinement, often for minor misbehavior and rule infractions; mail censorship; and re-stricted or absolute prohibitions on visitation and use of a tele-phone. Even more disturbing is the fact that there is evidence that the administrative and medical staff in some hospitals refuse to correct abuses documented by official authorities and only do so when threatened with legal action.*

Discussing the matter in 1992 at his office in Michigan, Schwartz said that on visits to more than a hundred hospitals with psychiatric units for children, he personally encountered instances of "rage reduction therapy—programs characterized by excessive use of restraint, handcuffs, solitary confinement," not to mention "very primitive behavior-modification regimes where kids start out in some cases wearing pajamas, and have to earn points so they can wear their own clothes, or even earn points to get better fed."

In 1985, the Mental Health Advocacy Office of Los Angeles County, looking into early complaints about for-profit psychiatric hospitals, issued a report about what it found in some of the chil-dren's wards:

One young patient was placed on 48-hour room isolation for accidentally bumping into a staff member in the cafeteria. The hospital records indicated that he was punished for engaging in "noncombative contact." . . .

While in the closed unit, a patient was assessed points for replying that he wanted "to go home" when asked for his hourly request. The records indicated that the staff felt that this was ". . . inappropriate reaction and sarcasm," warranting punishment. . . .

Patient C complained of being fined because, while playing the game Trivial Pursuit, he asked how the fictional character James Bond preferred his martinis (stirred, not shaken). A check of the [hospital's] fine point book confirmed his claim. On December 16 there was this entry: "Patient states 'How does James Bond like his martinis stirred?' " He was fined ten points for making a drug- and alcohol-related remark.

Again and again, whistle-blowers from corporate psychiatric hospitals complained about so-called "rage reduction therapy," widely employed to counter resistance. A standard reference book extolling the virtues of this technique is *High Risk: Children Without a Conscience,* by Ken Magid and Carole A. McKelvey, which refers to kids who resist as "trust bandits." Magid and McKelvey describe the therapy this way:

Basically, Rage Reduction Therapy involves physical holding and control of a patient who is confronted with his death-grip resistance to accepting love and acting responsibly. The therapy contains explosive dialogue as the psychopathic patient is encouraged to work through his unbelievable rage and anger while being forced to accept another's total control.

Rage Reduction Therapy is a moving emotional experience for the therapist, patient, and patient's parents.

Acknowledging that some critics have compared rage reduction therapy to brainwashing, the authors quote one leading proponent of the technique: "Some of these kids need their brains washed."

Another therapeutic technique is called chair therapy.

Like other behavior-modification methods, there is nothing new or "scientific" about it. In the United States, the chair as a therapeutic instrument for the insane was popularized in the early 1800s by Dr. Benjamin Rush, the founder of American psychiatry. Rush, who also espoused bloodletting as a way to relieve insanity, introduced into treatment a mechanical chair, which he called the Tranquilizer, to which a patient was strapped head and foot and encouraged to talk out problems while the physician evaluated sympathetically.

In 1990, Brenda Roberts, the energetic young college student who was employed to do marketing chores at Willowbrook Hospital in Texas, was utterly baffled when she took a subsequent part-time job at another psychiatric hospital a few months later and first saw "chair therapy." She would not identify the hospital because she was afraid doing so would mark her as a troublemaker and limit her career opportunities after college. But she talked willingly of her impressions.

"That first night I was there, all the kids were in chairs in the hallway," she recalled. "Some were facing the wall; some were facing the hallway. One girl in particular was crying; I approached her, asked her if she was okay, and at that time an employee came up to me and said, 'You don't speak to the kids whenever they're in chair.' And then I found out later than they're 'in chair' a lot of the time. The only time they spoke to staff members as far as discussing or expressing their feelings or anything going on with them was done in groups—it was very strict and very regulated. Anytime they were not in groups they were in the chair. . . . They ate in their chairs."

The food was often cold, but complaints were discouraged. In fact, talking itself was frowned on. "They couldn't look down the hallway right or left or they were given test marks." A "test mark," she explained, was like a demerit. "If you got five test marks, you got twenty-four hours chair. That meant you'd turn the chair around and face the wall."

Parents evidently weren't aware that their children were spending so much time in an activity that was billed as therapy but looked to her very much like punishment. "I don't ever remember a parent being on the unit. If a parent came to visit, the kid was removed from the unit, with a staff member accompanying them to the dining room. They visited with their parents there and then returned to the unit."

Brenda tried to just do her job and go home, but she was bothered by the way patients were treated. One night, she saw a young woman come in for counseling "to find out if she needed to be an inpatient." The hapless woman "ended up signing the papers to be admitted, but she changed her mind before she was taken to the unit." This made the hospital admissions staff unhappy. "They called a code on her," Brenda said, meaning that security was notified. "Basically, several staff members showed up and said, You either go back to the unit or we'll take you back to the unit. She ended up staying."

However, Brenda ended up leaving. She quit her job.

In 1991, a young Fort Worth woman named Sharon Swinnea experienced chair therapy firsthand after she decided to seek treatment for an eating disorder. Her family doctor referred her to NME's Brookhaven Psychiatric Pavilion, where Sharon, who is also deaf, was told there was a unit just for young people with eating disorders. There wasn't. Instead, she found herself in a locked ward.

Sharon's mother, Evelyn, recalled, "We were not allowed to have a conversation. She was not allowed to call us; we were not allowed to call her." When Sharon's parents objected, they were told that their daughter could die if they did not follow instructions.

With a mixture of embarrassment and determination to see that it not happen to anyone else, Sharon described the experience to investigators in Texas:

> *After being admitted I was required to completely strip for what they called a "body search," and asked to remove all my jewelry. I was told this was a suicide precaution, but I wasn't there for that reason, and couldn't understand what was happening to me.*
>
> *I begged to use the telephone to call my parents in Fort Worth, but was told I didn't have phone privileges: "Only your doctor could grant you those rights." When I questioned the doctor, I found out I couldn't use the phone for any reason. I also would not be allowed visitors, a rule which lasted for over two months. I felt as though I was being punished for my eating disorder rather than being treated.*
>
> *Every day there was some new rule. If I sat and kicked my leg, I was accused of "purposeful exercise." I would get placed in leather restraints; they would lock my legs to a chair for four to six hours at a time. If they caught me biting my fingernails they said it was "self-destructive" behavior and I was again placed in the leather restraints . . .*
>
> *Two weeks after I was admitted they had my parents come for a meeting where they were supposed to discuss my treatment plan, but instead it turned into a meeting of false accusations and insults to my parents. They told them that I was dying and they must agree to family therapy to help me. It scared them to death. Of course, they would do anything to help me. At least they could see me, although they were not allowed to have any physical contact with me or to meet with me alone.*
>
> *You were supposed to be allowed the have a felt-tip pen and loose notebook paper. My mother brought me these items, but I found out that I wasn't allowed them. The doctor put me on a "behavioral reward system" and I had to pay earned tokens to use my pen for an hour at a time.*

According to the [treatment] plan, I was not allowed to ask questions. I had to rephrase everything I said so it wouldn't be in question form. I was not allowed off the carpet in the day room, or I lost a token. One day, I had more than my body could handle. I wanted to talk to my parents and see them—I felt so alone and afraid of everything. They refused to grant me any of what I asked. In desperation, I threatened to pull out the stomach tube. They called in the team of assistants that puts you in leather restraints, and despite the fact I let go of the tube and promised not to touch it, I was strapped to the bed. My arms were stretched out tight and my legs were spread apart and strapped down, and I was taken out for all of the other patients to see what happens when you disobey. I was locked in the restraints for more than 24 hours. . . .

The middle of March, after discovering I was out of insurance, I was finally released from Brookhaven.

Among the hundreds of cases of abuse documented by the National Association of Protection and Advocacy Systems is one involving a therapeutic technique guaranteed to work on a child. In 1992, the Kentucky office represented a ten-year-old boy who was forced to eat by a nurse who held a hypodermic needle over his head and threatened to inject him with it if he did not clean his plate.

Less ugly, but almost as baffling to some parents looking with mouths agape at bills for their children's treatment in psychiatric hospitals, were therapeutic techniques such as "dance therapy" and "psychodrama."

A Houston-area man said he was floored when he read over the bill he received from NME's Laurelwood Hospital, where his daughter had been treated for depression. On a single day, June 25, 1990, the bill listed charges for fifteen group therapy sessions (at $45 each), three dance therapy sessions ($45 each) two-counseling sessions ($57.50 each) and one individual therapy session

($120). On another day, the bill indicated fourteen group therapy sessions, three dance therapy sessions, two "group counseling" sessions, and one individual session. The man's employee health insurance paid the bills, which totaled over $41,000. "My daughter had been hospitalized for psychiatric care, with no intent or interest in training for Bolshoi Ballet," the man said incredulously.

Another bewildered parent, Ronald J. Kellis, scrutinized the bills for his daughter's treatment item by item, scowling at the seven-dollar pills, even though his insurance company had already sent the check.

In 1990, Kellis, an airline computer scientist, had pulled his adopted thirteen-year-old daughter out of Psychiatric Institute of Fort Worth, an NME facility that heavily marketed its adolescent treatment programs. The girl had been in for six months; Kellis removed her against the hospital's wishes because he didn't think she was getting any better.

"We couldn't get a straight answer from anybody. I kept saying, 'Hey guys, what progress are we making?' They'd say, 'Oh, we're making progress, don't worry about that.' We weren't running out of insurance money. There was no rush." Kellis figured that his company insurance benefits probably provided a disincentive to a speedy cure. "Very good insurance," he said. "Each member of the family was covered for up to $500,000."

The girl was the oldest of three siblings whom Kellis and his wife had adopted five years earlier. The kids had been "exposed to" abuse of all kinds while living with their natural parents. "We had been warned that they would have emotional problems, and they did," Kellis said.

The bill for the girl's hospitalization was "in excess of $180,000." Though the money didn't come out of his pocket, Kellis bristled at the charges and tried to interest his insurance company in challenging items like numerous $160-per-session charges for what he learned were "community meetings" between patients and floor staff that "appeared on what billing I could get my hands on as therapy sessions."

Kellis said he couldn't get answers to his questions about the charges, and the insurance company wasn't concerned. "I asked the insurance people what prerogatives I had to force communications from Psychiatric Institute to my wife and myself. They didn't really seem interested in helping me. I mean, there was no outward expression of, Well, we'll work with you."

Parents didn't necessarily have to agree to have a child admitted, if the prospective patient fit into the right categories and had good insurance.

Curtis Decker of NAPAS was taken with the case of one high school senior in San Diego, described by investigators as "bright" and "energetic," with a 4.0 grade-point average. But after an argument with a boyfriend, the girl was depressed enough to call a toll-free number for counseling. A private psychiatric hospital operated the phone service. After being asked a series of questions the girl was told to come to the hospital for an evaluation the next day. When she arrived, she was immediately admitted and "because she had indicated [in questioning] that she had thought of suicide, the [hospital] was legally able to hold her for three days" without her or her parents' consent, Decker said. It took a Superior Court order to get her out.

In another case, a fifteen-year-old girl was committed to a psychiatric hospital for twenty-eight days (the limit of her family insurance coverage), diagnosed as being "severely defiant" toward her parents. The crux of the problem, however, was that the girl was white and defying her parents by dating a black youth.

Nick Sahadi, a Texas psychiatric worker, recalled that parents frequently tricked kids into psychiatric hospitalization. "I saw teenagers that I would know ahead of time who were coming in who were being told they were going to the dentist, or they were going for a checkup, and they would bring them in, get them behind the locked doors, and then—they didn't know what was going on— and then they were told 'You're in a psychiatric hospital and this is where you're going to stay.' "

"And a lot of the children, a lot of the teenagers, that came in there . . . were there because their parents didn't want to have anything to do with them, their parents wanted them out. When I talked to these kids, a lot of these kids were in school, they weren't having any serious troubles with the law or anything like that, but their parents would bring them into the hospital and sometimes these kids would be in there for a year, living at the hospital. They were not psychotic or manic-depressive—usually they were diagnosed as something like 'conduct . . . behavior.' "

Horror stories surfaced from throughout the country. The Oklahoma Office of Juvenile System Oversight looked into abuses of children at private psychiatric hospitals in 1991 and 1992. Among the investigation's findings:

• In Ada, Oklahoma, Rolling Hills Hospital agreed to stop charging children patients $40 a day for "relaxation therapy" that the oversight agency found consisted solely of taped music played in the hall while patients prepared for bed. The hospital also agreed to discontinue the use of straitjackets on children after state regulators objected.
• At Community Psychiatric Centers' Southwind Hospital in Oklahoma City, the juvenile-oversight agency found that a psychiatrist displayed a pair of rusty pliers to threaten a five-year-old child with having his teeth pulled out. This psychiatrist also threatened to cut the boy's fingers off.
• At Great Plains Hospital in Lawton, Oklahoma, a teenage girl, nearing the end of her sixty-day hospitalization, was improperly kept in the hospital after a staff therapist got a last-minute extension of the girl's Medicaid insurance benefits. The girl was told she was a suicide risk, and was detained over her

mother's objection. To justify the extended hospitalization, the hospital stated that the girl "suddenly got worse" a few days before her scheduled discharge. But the juvenile agency found that actually the girl's reaction was the direct result of being told she couldn't leave. "This patient's treatment was not only disjointed and unprofessional," said the agency's report, "but it potentially lessened this child's ability to trust adults who provide direction and guidance."

• At High Pointe psychiatric hospital in Oklahoma City, the agency concluded, teenage patients who were forced to eat in the unit due to privilege restrictions were required to do chair time, yielding the perception that they were required to "earn" their lunches; whole units were punished for the infractions of a single patient; and patients' therapy sessions with psychiatrists were sporadic, sometimes lasting less than ten minutes.

Gossip and water-cooler cynicism thrive in any hospital environment, but usually the staff keeps its own counsel. But in many psychiatric hospitals, on-ward professionals such as nurses and counselors openly derided the physicians they saw blatantly hustling the system and profitably acquiescing in hospital management's pressure to fully exploit insurance benefits, with little regard for patient care.

One patient nicknamed a Laurelwood Hospital psychiatrist Hundred-Dollar-a-Handshake. The monicker came from the knowledge that a patient's only contact with this physician usually was a handshake and a few words. So-called group therapy sessions were derided openly as "mob therapy" because they were often conducted with twenty and more kids in attendance. One sixteen-year-old girl, committed as a manic-depressive for an unusually long eighteen months under her parents' liberal insurance plan, finally contacted a young man who agreed to marry her so that she could declare herself an adult and get out of the hospital. "We never consummated the marriage," the girl said.

A former Laurelwood unit director recalled that adolescent discharges were planned to the day upon arrival, on the basis of the maximum number of days for which insurance would pay. "The absolutely worst thing you could have on your unit was an unplanned discharge." A PIA spokesman explained that patient stays were a compromise between what the hospital believed the patient needed and what the insurer would pay. "In more than ninety percent of cases, the insurance company or a representative of the company is directly involved in treatment planning. The insurance company will dictate the length of stay. We'll say we want twenty-eight days to treat, and the insurance company says it will pay for only twenty-one."

Similarly, NME said in 1991 that for 90 percent of its patients in Texas, "their insurer or the insurer's representative conducts an independent clinical review of both the medical necessity for and the appropriateness of treatment."

Meanwhile, as federal, state, and county budgets dried up for community mental-health treatment, concerned public mental-health officials lamented what Barbara Demming Lurie, of the Los Angeles County health department, called the irony of "an acute shortage" of services for adolescents without private health insurance. "The county has to turn away many severely disturbed youngsters for lack of resources while kids who may not need or want inpatient psychiatric treatment are getting it in the private sector," she said.

Weary workers at public and nonprofit mental-health centers sometimes are able accommodate some troublesome kids after the private hospitals dump them, "where the private psychiatric hospital industry has drained the family's insurance benefits," said Mitch Weynand, the director of a public crisis center and youth shelter in Austin, Texas. He said that when seeing such a kid arrive with overnight bag, shelter workers turn to each other with a standard joke: "Oh, he's been cured today. His parents' insurance ran out."

CHAPTER EIGHT

....

BY 1991, AFTER A DECADE OF LOBBYING AND MEDIA PROMOTION by mental-health and substance-abuse interests, more than 95 percent of all U.S. companies employing more than a hundred people had benefit plans providing coverage for alcoholism and drug-abuse treatment. This was more than double the number of companies that had such benefits in 1983, according to the *Monthly Labor Review.*

The fortunes of the psychiatric-hospital business closely tracked this largesse, a trend vividly illustrated by the fact that the number of exclusively psychiatric private hospitals in the United States doubled, to 444, in the period 1984 to 1988, with concurrent growth in the number of general medical hospitals offering expanded in-patient psychiatric-treatment programs.

According to data from the federal Center for Mental Health Services, from 1983 through 1988 (the last year for which figures are available), per capita expenditures on private psychiatric hospitals more than doubled. The number of private psychiatric beds per 100,000 of civilian population more than doubled in the same period. And so did the rate of inpatient admissions.

In 1981, at the onset of this amazing era during which psychiatry strove with great success to insert itself into the routine process of

American medical care, one of the towering entrepreneurs of the industry anticipated the rosy future. William A. Fickling, Jr., a founder and the president of Charter Medical, the leading corporation in the psychiatric industry, used the company's annual report to log his predictions as the pilot of a high-flying business with nothing but blue skies ahead. It had been just one year since Charter had made the most important strategic decision in its corporate history, electing not to build any more general hospitals but to instead refocus on psychiatric hospitals. Fickling wrote:

> *Tragically, as addictive disease becomes increasingly exposed to the light of understanding and compassion, evidence mounts that the problem of substance abuse may be reaching epidemic proportions. Alcoholism, a disease once thought to be confined to a relatively small segment of the adult population, appears to be afflicting adolescents, and even children, in alarming numbers.*

The following year, Fickling enthusiastically told shareholders: "We are in the midst of the most active psychiatric hospital construction program in our highly competitive industry," with three new hospitals opened in 1982 and four more scheduled to open in 1983.

> *Perhaps the most disturbing aspect of addictive disease—and of mental illness—is that frequently it is ignored or covered up by the individual or family, despite the fact that treatment often is effective. Recovery necessitates a recognition of the problem by the person, and a commitment by the patient and his or her family to work productively through the difficulty. If hospitalization is indicated, it takes the experience of a compassionate and understanding physician and professional staff to help the patient set meaningful goals and to achieve them.*

140

Happily for Charter's stockholders, hospitalization appears to have been indicated very often. By 1987, when Fickling and some top associates startled Wall Street with an announcement that they were taking the company private in a whopping $1.5 billion management buyout, Charter was setting the pace in the furiously profitable but increasingly debt-burdened psychiatric industry. Charter had gone from five psychiatric hospitals in 1977 to sixty-three a decade later. In 1987, those sixty-three psychiatric hospitals generated $559 million in revenues, a delectable 80 percent of which came from the most highly prized source, commercial health insurance. (Another 12 percent came from Medicare, the federal insurance for old people, and only a tiny 4 percent came from Medicaid, the state and federal program for insuring the poor.) During one period of this spree, Charter employed seven senior executives charged with opening new hospitals.

The Recovery Era had joined forces with the Therapeutic State. As it was everywhere else in the economy of the eighties, it was party time in the psychiatric industry.

The term "Therapeutic State" was popularized in the early sixties by a group of iconoclastic New York psychiatrists led by Thomas S. Szasz, who defined it as the political manifestation of psychiatry's inherent impulse to acquire extralegal authority to impose behavioral control. In the Therapeutic State, as Szasz and his cohorts saw it, the medical model is used to broadly define certain behaviors as diseases, opening the way for intervention by "medicalized" psychiatry, in the same way biological medicine intervened to combat diseases like cholera.

In the late seventies, with a burst of what would become relentless media promotion of self-help bromides and addiction-cure nostrums, the imperatives of the Recovery Era were laid atop the Therapeutic State, inducing ever-growing numbers of people to countenance medical and other therapeutic intervention in ever-widening areas of behavior. The result, depending on your point of view, might be considered "expensive pseudomedical therapies

[that] exacerbate the problems they ostensibly attack and are a step toward totalitarianism," as clinical psychologist Stanton Peele put it pointedly in his 1989 book, *Diseasing of America: Addiction Treatment Out of Control*. Or, as the gurus of the self-help and recovery industries insist, the result was a healthy awareness that nearly every person in American society was addicted or otherwise psychologically crippled—if not by booze and pills, then by depression, stress, overeating, low self-esteem, overwork, lechery, sadness, incompetence, obnoxiousness, and an inexhaustible list of other conditions that only peripherally included certifiable lunacy.

Szasz once cited an impression Charles Dickens reported in 1842 after his first visit to America: "Instead of simply acknowledging their wrongdoing," Dickens wrote, "Americans prefer to deny it with a dramatic gesture of undoing."

The Recovery Era gesture was dramatic indeed. During the eighties, the revenues of U.S. private psychiatric hospitals—not counting the thousands of psychiatric facilities in general hospitals—surged from less than $1 billion to nearly $7 billion.

Free-standing psychiatric hospitals are relatively inexpensive to run, not being places that require large acute-care medical staffs or expensive labs and diagnostic equipment. Their profit structures are more closely related to hotels', with nearly all of the revenue coming from daily room rates (affiliated psychiatrists bill separately, like consulting specialists in a general hospital). They also have few concerns about getting their money, since they seldom accept patients without full insurance. At private psychiatric hospitals, for example, about 85 percent of revenue comes from private insurance, as opposed to less than 60 percent in for-profit general hospitals. Almost all of the rest comes from Medicare insurance, and a small percentage from Medicaid.

Mental health policy, drafted in the eighties by federal officials with close ties to the biopsychiatric industry, supports the psychiatric-hospital industry's goals for growth. In 1988, the National Institute of Mental Health publicized its findings that in any given

six-month period, 19.1 percent of adult Americans met the diagnostic criteria for mental illness (and over a lifetime, 32.2 percent
did). The report described a veritable cornucopia of anxiety disorders, phobias, panic disorders, obsessive-compulsive disease,
addictions, depressions, and manias. With barely concealed glee,
the National Association of Private Psychiatric Hospitals declared
in its annual report for 1988: "This means that one in three adults
can expect to have a diagnosable mental illness or a serious drug
or alcohol abuse problem at some point in their lifetime." Not to
mention the children: "A study for the Children's Defense Fund
in 1982 showed that at least three million children in this country
are seriously mentally ill"—that is, mentally ill for more than one
year, the association said in its annual survey for 1989. In all, "as
many as 14 million children and adolescents experience mental
disorders, many of which persist into adulthood."

The association did lament that "lack of adequate insurance still
presents a significant barrier to psychiatric care for some 37 million
uninsured or underinsured Americans."

The psychiatric hospitals prospered on what has been called the
"legalization of expectations" brought out by the marketing of the
Recovery Era. Starting in the late 1970s, and buoyed by a spirit
of personal responsibility for maintaining good health, Americans
were encouraged to embrace new treatments for mental health,
especially in the areas such as drug and alcohol addiction and
personal and family unhappiness. Areas of behavior that had traditionally been stashed away in family closets were suddenly openly
confronted. As celebrities such as Betty Ford and cocaine-addled
basketball stars issued ringing testimonials (and often accepted
salaries for doing so), inpatient treatment in profit-making psychiatric and substance-abuse facilities became not only acceptable, but
in some circles actually *fashionable*. If money could buy the best
of anything in the 1980s, why not the best recovery?

New benefits under employee insurance coverage were hailed
as marking the advent of a new era in pro-active mental health

care, the benchmark of nothing less than a bold national recovery program. In an American tradition not acted out on this scale since the days of the Great Society, America identified a problem and threw money at it. Private enterprise, freed in the Reagan years from excessive governmental regulation, rushed into place to capture the vast beckoning market.

The psychiatric hospital industry, which soon became a favorite of Wall Street, augmented the marketing and promotion with effective lobbying state by state and corporation by corporation to have new areas of psychiatric care covered by employee insurance. To a national medical bill that had been soaring out of control, a huge new charge was now added for comprehensive psychiatric care—at least, for those with employee insurance. Corporate health-insurance providers added benefits for an astonishing array of addiction, crisis, and counseling programs.

A 1986 survey of three hundred major U.S. employers by the American Psychiatric Association found that nearly half of them provided inpatient coverage for hospital psychiatric treatment on the same basis as for any other illness. That percentage grew steadily higher over succeeding years.

Coverage for alcohol- and substance-abuse treatment rose especially sharply; by 1990, an estimated 96 percent of employee health-insurance plans provided inpatient treatment for alcoholism, and 93 percent covered alcohol and drug treatment—up from 68 and 61 percent respectively in 1985, according to a national survey sponsored by the Employee Benefits Research Institute.

By the end of the decade, twenty-nine states would actually mandate that employers provide inpatient coverage for mental-health care; forty-one would require coverage for alcohol-abuse treatment and twenty-seven for drug abuse, according to a survey commissioned by the Health Insurance Association of America. At the same time, the psychiatric industry had successfully introduced the notion of "dual diagnosis" treatment into the health-care system. For example, someone diagnosed with alcohol addiction might also be diagnosed as suffering from a concomitant disorder of depression, opening up two separate categories for insurance reimbursement.

Yet equally remarkable was the credence that newspapers and television—anxious to fill newly devoted columns and interminable hours of programming with "lifestyle" and "personal health"—gave to claims by the psychiatric industry, which maintains that sixty million Americans—including twelve million children—require psychiatric services, the overwhelming majority of which are provided through inpatient hospitalization.

The costs of untreated mental illness and substance abuse are said to be far higher than the costs to pay the psychiatric industry to "cure" them. In the mid-eighties, the National Association of Private Psychiatric Hospitals came up with a precise figure—complete with decimal point—for the costs to U.S. business of mental illness and drug and alcohol abuse: $237.6 billion a year.

(In *Diseasing of America*, Stanton Peele notes that in its 1972 report to Congress, the National Institute on Alcohol Abuse and Alcoholism estimated that alcoholism alone cost the U.S. economy $15 billion that year. Ten years later, Peele points out, despite many billions of dollars in federal spending to combat alcoholism, the same agency reported that the cost had increased almost eightfold, to $116 billion. In 1990, the federal government itself spent $5 billion on the so-called War on Drugs. Yet Recovery Era authorities have recently been estimating that as many as two hundred million Americans currently are suffering from the effects of their or someone else's substance abuse, leading Peele and other skeptics to wonder, if these assertions are true, what exactly all that money bought.)

By the end of the decade, a whole subculture of recovery had come to maturity. In a 1991 *Harper's* magazine article entitled "Victims, All?" author David Reiff asked:

> *Imagine a country in which millions of apparently successful people nonetheless have come to believe that they are really lost souls . . . where countless adults allude matter-of-factly to their "inner children" who, they say, lie wounded and in desperate need of relief with the wreckage of their grown-up selves. Imagine the celebrities and opinion-makers among these people talking nightly on TV and weekly in the magazines not about their triumphs but about their victimization, not about their power and fame, but about their addictions and childhood persecutions.*
>
> *Imagine that this belief in abused "inner children" dragging down grown-up men and women has become so widespread as to exert considerable influence over the policies of such supposedly practical bodies as corporations, public hospitals and boards of education.*

Charles J. Sykes, author of *A Nation of Victims: The Decay of the American Character*, takes note of a man who, having embezzled money and lost it in Atlantic City casinos, sued to win back his job because he was a victim of "compulsive gambling syndrome," and of a school administrator, fired for constantly missing classes, who calls himself a victim of "compulsive lateness syndrome."

Writing in *The New York Times*, Sykes noted that the National Association of Sexual Addiction Problems estimates that between 10 percent and 15 percent of the U.S. population are "addicted" to sex. More than 20 million Americans are "addicted" to gambling, says another interest group, the National Council on Compulsive Gambling. A leader of the "co-dependency" movement estimates that more than two hundred million Americans suffer from the effects of abusive, addicted "or merely critical" parents. Sykes laments the rise of "dysfunctional and aggrieved populace" that has caused "national gridlock" in its "irresistible search for someone or something to blame colliding with an unwillingness to accept responsibility."

By the nineties, the language of the Recovery Era permeated American society. In a 1992 *New Yorker* profile of television talk show host Jay Leno, Peter J. Boyer recounts that two NBC executives arrived unannounced at Leno's home and told him he had to fire his longtime producer, who was disliked by network brass. Leno's relationship with the producer had become an "addiction," said Warren Littlefield, who was then the president of NBC Entertainment. Indeed, Littlefield announced to the astonished Leno: "This is an intervention."

"Psychobabble" from the Recovery Era has even become a problem for normally easygoing veterans of groups like Alcoholics Anonymous, some of whom now openly grumble about the influx of new members whose problem seems to be less alcoholism than chronic narcissism. "I don't even go to the meetings anymore because of these people. They never shut up about themselves. Most of them belong to two or three twelve-step groups," said one longtime AA member in 1992. "It's enough to drive you back to drink."

In "Don't Blame Me," a 1991 story in *New York* magazine, John Taylor wrote: "When Richard Berendzen, the former president of American University, resigned last year after admitting to having made obscene phone calls from his office, a doctor named Kenneth Grundfast argued in the *Washington Post* that Berendzen deserved public sympathy because he was a victim of an obsessive-compulsive disorder which often is "caused more by abnormal DNA sequences within an individual's chromosomes than by . . . moral lapses."

Moral lapses, however, are not usually covered by health insurance. But call them "abnormal DNA sequences within an individual's chromosomes," as the psychiatric industry has come to do, and the check is in the mail.

This is the main reason the psychiatric industry grew, and in the process coopted a large segment of the profession of psychiatry, whose complicity is required to fill out the medical charts for in-surance review. As "medicine," psychiatry is now overwhelmingly skewed toward hospitals. Why? As the bank robber Willie Sutton once replied when asked why he robbed banks, "That's where all the money is."

During the eighties, while state legislatures were besieged with lobbyists from the psychiatric industry, consumer medical groups tried to point out that the sweeping mandates requiring mental-health and addiction coverage by employer health-insurance pol-icies were in fact a primary cause of dwindling access to health care for all, as well as an important factor in soaring overall health-insurance costs.

"Mandated benefits are very often a response to special interest groups and perceived needs," Emily Crandall, a vice president of Guardian Life of New York, told *Psychiatric News*. "Most people who do not have health insurance do not have it because they flat-out cannot afford the various products we are mandated to sell in various states."

Waving the banner of the Recovery Era, the psychiatric industry was very successful at modifying the hospital-building restrictions most states used to prevent an oversupply of hospital beds, equip-ment, and clinical services. These restrictions, often called certif-icate-of-need laws, disappeared altogether in twelve states from 1983 to 1990, and were substantially relaxed in many others. Mean-while, the Reagan administration eliminated federal funding for state health-care-planning agencies (the offices that usually super-vised hospital construction), and abolished regulations restricting federal health-care spending in those states with relaxed certificate-of-need legislation.

Psychiatric hospitals aggressively took advantage of the oppor-tunities. By the end of the 1980s, states without certificate-of-need laws had an average number of for-profit psychiatric beds that was 33 percent higher than the average in regulated states, according to *Modern Healthcare*, a hospital trade magazine. Charter Medical operates most of its hospitals in states without certificate-of-need legislation.

Texas is a good example. In 1985, Texas legislators, responding to coordinated lobbying from psychiatric organizations and the hospital industry, and reacting to allegations that the existing system was corrupt and favored entrenched hospital interests, did away with certificate-of-need requirements. That year, there were thirty private psychiatric hospitals in the state. Seven years later, there were ninety. All over the country throughout the second half of the eighties, the for-profit psychiatric hospitals all reported surprisingly uniform average stays, of about twenty-eight days—which happened to coincide with the average number of days a year of inpatient psychiatric treatment provided by employee health-insurance policies. Patients "were cured miraculously on the day their insurance benefits ran out," State Senator Mike Moncrief said after he and his colleagues began to look into reports of profiteering in Texas. "Twenty-eight days seemed to be the magic number."

Moncrief recalled the days when Texas had a certificate-of-need law regulating hospital construction: "You used to have to justify why you needed those beds." But the rapidly expanding psychiatric-hospital corporation spoke the langauge of the 1980s: money and competitive edge. "Unfortunately, it became a political Super Bowl of sorts," Moncrief said. Whether a community actually needed more psychiatric beds wasn't the point—new demand could be created with marketing. "It became a question of economic development—more jobs, more tax base."

In the meantime, community crisis centers, low-cost outpatient drug and alcohol facilities, and even psychotherapists were squeezed out in the rush into the medical model. Treatment for severe mental illness—a debilitation usually associated with poverty—is languishing because there is no money in it. In the years of private psychiatric hospitals' initial growth spree from 1974 to

1984, there was a 53 percent reduction in the number of beds in state mental hospitals, with concurrent reductions in availability of community-based public mental-heath services.

According to Robert P. Stewart, the president of the National Association of Social Workers: "There is a fundamental difference in the application of free-market principles to products and services in the usual realms of commerce, as contrasted with their application to services responding to human suffering and distress. The extraordinary vulnerability of many consumers of mental-health services opens the potential for exploitation almost beyond imagining."

In his 1992 warning about the "medical industrial complex" in *The Atlantic*, Dr. Relman, the former editor of the *New England Journal of Medicine*, said: "The first step must be to gain a firm consensus on what we value in health care and what kind of a medical profession we want."

CHAPTER NINE

....

THERE WAS LITTLE DOUBT ABOUT THE MEDICAL AGENDA AT PSY-chiatric Institutes of America, PIA, which was what NME called its prized psychiatric hospital division before the name was dropped like a hot potato in 1992. At PIA's national and regional marketing seminars—which some participants thought resembled motivational sessions for door-to-door vacuum-cleaner sales—the PIA Marketeers, as they were called, sang songs that had lyrics that celebrated the joys of keeping beds full with paying customers and outsmarting the competition.

For those who were with it, marketing and sales meetings could be a jolly time. Sales videos exhorted the Marketeers to join in on sing-a-longs, one of which featured a ditty, sung to the tune of "Looking for Love in All the Wrong Places," whose chorus went:

> I was lookin' for patients in all the wrong places;
> Slummin' for admissions in noninsured places.

Except for the few grouches who muttered that this was not an appropriate way to approach the psychiatric hospitalization of adults and children, the Marketeers knew that they had a lot to sing about. Profits were piling up at record levels, and the future was golden;

every employee, doctor and receptionist alike, was expected to be a member of the sales force, singing lustily with the choir triumphant as the eighties roared.

Of course, psychiatric hospitals certainly were not alone in the health-care industry in embracing the convictions of modern marketing and advertising. By 1991, all U.S. hospitals—general and psychiatric—were spending about $2.97 billion a year on marketing and advertising, according to a survey by Quality Expectations, a health-care marketing firm. Hospitals are major U.S. economic forces; forty cents of every health-care dollar goes to a hospital, according to the trade journal *Modern Healthcare*. (This figure does not include the money doctors receive.) With at least 40 percent of all public and private hospital beds occupied by psychiatric and substance-abuse patients, mental health is by far the largest single revenue source.

Hospital marketing and advertising hit full force in the mid-eighties, as the psychiatric industry geared up to fill all the new beds it was creating, while the already overbuilt general hospital business scurried to stem the sharp drop in occupancy rates caused by stricter federal Medicare rules.

Frequently brandishing slogans and brand-name logos with the verve of fast-food chains, many hospitals became marketing-driven enterprises. In their executive suites, hometown faces with at least some background in community-based health care were replaced by corporate transplants who more often than not had spent their careers in such fields as hotel development or restaurant franchising. Even the language changed, with terms such as "showroom traffic" and "product niche" applied for the first time to hospital medicine. "This is 'Burger Wars' in health care," crowed one Chicago advertising-agency executive in 1984, explaining that hospitals were learning that they had to offer customers their own version of "Do you want it flame-broiled or fried?" A former admissions counselor at one Arizona hospital recalled that the staff referred to patients with insurance coverage for full psychiatric care as Cadillacs and those with partial coverage as Hondas.

By the nineties, as the systemic abuses started to come to light, Senator Moncrief of Texas exclaimed in wonder, "Marketing heretofore unknown to man is being utilized" to sell psychiatric treatment. Added Elizabeth Hubbard, a former marketing director for a private psychiatric hospital in the Southwest: "If you've got a wart on your butt, they'll find ten people to develop a psychiatric program for it."

"Mental heath care depends on sales," Gary Kagan, an Illinois marketing specialist, told the trade journal *Hospitals* in 1986. His firm, Horizon Health Management Company, introduced mental-health-care programs with brand names, such as "Balance" to treat eating disorders, and "ReNew" for chemical dependency.

It isn't clear how much of total hospital marketing outlay is accounted for by psychiatric hospitals, but it is clear that they, by far the most aggressive marketers in health care, had strong motivation to fill their beds with paying customers.

An illustration of that motivation comes from statistics tucked into the minutiae of financial data reported by Hospital Corporation of America (HCA), the national chain of both general and psychiatric hospitals, in its 1991 annual disclosure to the Securities and Exchange Commission. Side by side, the figures help to explain why the psychiatric industry is so eager to advertise itself with the gusto of a motel chain:

In 1991, HCA's seventy-four general hospitals received just 18 percent of their total revenue from patients' basic room-and-board charges. The bulk of general-hospital revenue came from ancillary charges such as inpatient radiology and other lab fees, operating rooms and the pharmacy (56 percent), and outpatient services (18 percent).

On the other hand, HCA's fifty-four psychiatric hospitals depended on room-and-board charges for 77 percent of total revenues in 1991. Pharmacy charges came in a distant second. Outpatient revenue was almost insignificant.

Advertising and marketing for psychiatric patients intensified toward the end of the eighties, with the market beginning to look saturated and with employers cutting back on the number of days of inpatient mental-health treatment they would pay for. By 1991, the average length of stay for a patient at HCA psychiatric hospitals was eighteen days, down significantly from 25.5 days in 1987. But more patients were being brought in to fill the void. The total number of people admitted to HCA psychiatric hospitals increased 10 percent in 1990 and another 6 percent in 1991.

In their relentless drive for market share, corporate psychiatric hospitals worked to establish profitable relationships with community providers of free or low-cost mental-health and substance-abuse care, who had access to a pool of potential patients who could be evaluated for insurance coverage. Often, the lure was an occasional free bed for the critical charity case, in exchange for a steady supply of referrals of potential paying customers. Frank Glover, a former coordinator of a state-funded outpatient drug-treatment facility, was given routine free lunches and tours of the hospital. As government funding dried up in the eighties, nonprofit and community treatment centers constantly scrounged for free beds for acute cases. "In all cases, the [hospital] marketing representatives implied that the more insured patients referred would increase my chances of obtaining a charity bed for one of our program clients," Glover said.

Early on in the Recovery Era, a compliant news media, eager to publicize testimonials by "recovering" celebrities such as Betty Ford, helped to accustom health-care consumers—and insurance providers—to the notion that expensive in-hospital treatment regimens were the best way to deal with problems like alcohol and drug abuse, mood disorders such as depression, and a wide range of behavioral and situational problems. Thanks to this onslaught of promotional publicity, for the first time large numbers of patients began arriving through referrals from people other than physicians.

Besides Mrs. Ford, other celebrities who helped to establish this system included John Phillips, a singer with The Mamas and the Papas, and his daughter MacKenzie, a television actress. Both were treated at Fair Oaks in New Jersey and heavily promoted the hospital's programs with national publicity. NME hired Patty Duke, another actress, to travel and lecture as "a role model" for its psychiatric programs, and even named a wing at one California hospital after her: the Patty Duke Center for Depression. Cathy Rigby, a former Olympic gymnast, made commercials in the mid-eighties promoting an inpatient eating-disorder program run by College Hospital, a private facility near Los Angeles. Comprehensive Care Corporation, a California-based corporation that owned psychiatric and alcohol- and drug-abuse facilities around the country, hired Billy Carter, brother of the former president, and Dallas Cowboys linebacker Thomas "Hollywood" Henderson to promote its inpatient substance-abuse programs.

Remedial marketing was used for damage control on those rare occasions when reliable news-media sources debunked claims that supported the foundation of profit-making hospital psychiatry. One virtually unassailable tenet was the well-established idea, often publicized by such sources as television talk shows and women's magazines, that as many as *half* of the young women in America suffer from bulimia, a disorder for which many for-profit psychiatric hospitals market inpatient treatment. In 1988, *The New York Times* reported that, according to new medical studies, "Widespread reports of a dangerous epidemic of the eating disorder bulimia are vastly overstated. . . . Researchers using a rigorous definition of the disorder, say they have found that it is rare, even among college women, the group considered most susceptible. . . . The studies also indicate that, contrary to many reports, the incidence of the disorder is not increasing."

"We were told to be ready to march out at a moment's notice to rebut that story, but the truth is, no one really paid any attention to it, because our marketing was so incessant," recalled a nurse from a central Florida hospital that still heavily advertises its eating-disorder program to the mothers of teenage girls. "Luckily, the local media ignored it."

According to a 1986 survey conducted for the psychiatric-hospital industry by a national marketing firm, only 8 percent of Americans then would have considered seeking help at a psychiatric facility for emotional problems. Obviously, referral sources needed to be established to address this recalcitrance. Clergy members, teachers, employee counselors, and others who are exposed to confidential psychological information about people could be enlisted to help move patients into the pipeline. "Clearly, a mental health facility can increase its market position by improving relations with these groups," a marketing specialist told a hospital-industry trade journal.

For the first time, marketing was effectively applied to health care not only to promote existing services, but also to create demand for "new product." As part of their promotional strategy, psychiatric hospitals routinely augment advertising and other marketing activities by publicizing themselves as regional centers for "lifestyle" information. Over coffee and cake at many hospitals, hundreds of people—potential customers all—attend advertised weekly lectures on stress, time management, parenting, and a wide range of other topics, most of which have corresponding treatment programs.

Palmview Hospital in Lakeland, Florida, devised a promotion called "House Calls—An Old-Fashioned Idea at Home in the '90s," which borrowed a "social networking" marketing strategy more often associated with home-product sales. The hospital invites a potential hostess or host to select a topic from a list of subjects such as depression, anxiety, "loss and grieving," obsessive-compulsive disorders, "marriage enrichment," overeating, dating, and "Satanism & Teens." The hostess or host then provides the hospital with names and addresses of about twenty-five friends who might be interested in attending. The hospital sends out invitations, and on the appointed date provides "a physician or other mental health professional" to lecture the group in the comfortable confines of the home of a friend, who receives a twenty-dollar gift certificate for hosting the soirée. The hospital, in turn, gets a roomful of potential patients—people already well disposed toward the speaker and interested enough in the subject to listen to a sales pitch—as well as a network of future potential hostesses and hosts.

"I have seen that kind of marketing only one other place—Tupperware parties," said a disgusted former staff counselor. "But at least you know what you're buying with Tupperware."

Behind the scenes, however, the marketing is sometimes not so congenial. A nurse at one psychiatric hospital said that hospital administrators "tape-recorded [employee] telephone calls and rated their employees on the their ability to persuade patients to come in for a free evaluation, which would hopefully lead to an admission."

One of the most profitable ways for psychiatric hospitals to identify "motivated buyers," as marketing departments refer to people distressed enough to inquire about treatment, is with crisis hot lines. These are toll-free numbers, often listed in phone books and on billboards, that appear to offer free emergency help for people in emotional crisis, but sometimes are actually a direct pipeline into a psychiatric hospital's marketing department. Some are operated by third-party agencies that receive referral fees—the fees that cantankerous investigators in Texas insist on calling bounties—for each insured patient who is admitted.

More even than "Books as Hooks," the hot-line subterfuge riled Texas lawmakers when they began to delve into the practices of psychiatric hospitals after Senator Tejeda's office brought Jeramy Harrell's case to light.

Senator Moncrief, for one, was astounded by the way some of the hot lines operated.

"A 1-800 suicide hot line advertised in the San Antonio telephone book refers callers to a 1-900 number, where they make two dollars a minute off your call while you're deciding whether to take your life!" Moncrief exclaimed with astonishment in 1991. "What is happening in Texas, I guarantee you is happening in every other state in this country."

He was right, of course.

Crisis hot lines, promoted in big type in the Yellow Pages, on billboards, and on television, seldom stress (and often don't even mention) the fact that many are referral sources for psychiatric hospitals as well as community nonprofit counseling services. One toll-free hot-line number operated out of Long Beach, California, advertised all over the country for suicide prevention and depression counseling. After establishing whether they had insurance, it referred callers to the admissions systems of various private psychiatric hospitals—and pocketed a referral fee for each.

The same service—the one Moncrief was shaking his head over—in addition to referrals to free programs, listed a 900-number where callers who did not have adequate insurance for referral to a private hospital were charged $2.50 a minute to receive alternate referral information on county and other public help—and then sent on their way.

"Telemarketing," as the hot-line strategies are known, came to hospital psychiatry in the 1970s, at the height of public alarm over drug use by young people. The hot-line business, though energized by the introduction of automated and computerized telephone systems, has always depended mightily on the ability of a live operator to get the caller headed to the hospital's admission office as quickly as possible.

Comprehensive Care Corporation operated a national toll-free hot line, keyed to television advertising, that received more than 31,000 calls in 1985, "half of which were patched back to individual hospitals," *Advertising Age* reported. The company said the hot line was a factor in a third of the 62,000 admissions to its facilities in 1985. By 1986, Comprehensive Care had hired a major ad agency, DDB/Needham Worldwide, to develop a hot-line–oriented cocaine-treatment advertising campaign.

By the eighties, telephone hot lines had evolved into a crucial marketing tool in many areas of health care. For example, the National Cancer Institute introduced its "Cancer Information Service" toll-free hot line in 1983. "Its call load doubled to 500,000 between 1983 and 1985," *Advertising Age* reported in 1986, adding that according to a study, nearly a quarter of all hot-line callers subsequently "made appointments with physicians, clinics or hospitals."

One of the most successful hot lines was 800-COCAINE, founded in 1983 by Dr. Mark S. Gold, a prominent psychiatrist who was director of research for NME's Fair Oaks hospitals in both New Jersey and Florida. Gold, who served as a consultant on drug policy for the Reagan administration, is the author of several books on addiction and mental health, including *The Good News About Depression: Cures and Treatment in the New Age of Psychiatry*, which heralded the triumph of biopsychiatry in the 1980s, asserting that "the biopsychiatric approach has become *the* way at many of the best psychiatric centers in the country."

NME signaled its growing interest in telephone marketing in its 1984 annual report, which boasted of national "Counseline" phone recordings that provided information on "personal, emotional and mental health problems." The next year, Chairman Richard Eamer told stockholders about the successes of new "major outreach programs, such as the '800-COCAINE' hot line, which persons in crisis throughout the nation may call on for intervention and referral information."

Advertised nationally on billboards and in telephone Yellow Pages as a "confidential not-for-profit service," 800-COCAINE had been controversial almost from its inception. Some critics charged that callers were not always aware that they were contacting a service operated by a for-profit psychiatric facility, even though operators usually identified the hot line as "a service of Fair Oaks Hospital." Although Fair Oaks paid the hot line's bills and provided its offices, the 800-COCAINE coordinator, Peter Gold, Mark Gold's cousin, described it as a public service that referred callers to various treatment outlets, including nonprofit ones. A hospital administrator said in 1987 that Fair Oaks in Delray Beach received only about "two or three patients a month" through referrals by 800-COCAINE.

The Miami Herald reported in 1987 that Florida callers to 800-COCAINE were always asked about their insurance coverage. "If the caller had insurance, he or she was directed to seek treatment at Fair Oaks Hospital in Delray Beach," the newspaper reported after conducting a two-week survey. Those asking for an alternative to Fair Oaks, which then charged $22,000 for a 28-day stay, were given the number of "an overburdened public-supported treatment facility [with] a three-to-four–week waiting list," the newspaper said.

Nationally, 800-COCAINE was reported to be logging 1,200 calls a day in 1986, and twice that number when promotions for cocaine addiction were placed on national television news programs.

In the eighties, another hospital company introduced a pioneering hot-line prrogram with a year-long newspaper advertising campaign that listed a phone number for callers to obtain a free booklet, "How to Handle a Mental Crisis." Calls were taken by counselors for a private psychiatric hospital in California. "Census rose considerably, and for the first time in the history of the facility, physicians came to us for referrals, instead of the reverse," the head of the hospital's ad agency said.

The key to all this is a highly motivated sales staff. Private psychiatric hospitals approached the challenge with the zeal of evangelists. At some hospital sales meetings, employees were even expected to stand up and testify.

James Hutchison, a psychologist who ran the adolescent outpatient program at NME's Baywood Hospital in Texas for two years until 1989, recalled weekly marketing meetings "conducted in the atmosphere of a booster rally, with prizes for the employees with the most marketing points." At Baywood, he said, "every employee, from groundskeeper to program director, from office secretary to nurse, was obliged to conduct weekly marketing calls." Every employee had a quota, and "a computer check was run regularly to identify employees who initiated admissions." Prizes for the best performers included free pizzas and theater and sports tickets.

Hutchison had no doubt that revenue was everything: "Program directors of inpatient units were required to account for any discharges of patients with hospital stays of less than one month after admission. 'Early' discharges, defined as patients with insurance coverage who were discharged in less than one month, were strongly discouraged."

He described inpatient revenue as the preferred treatment, with outpatient programs such as the one he ran designed largely as "feeder channels to inpatient programs." Furthermore, community-based "outreach clinics" offering free services had one basic mission: "to convert inquiries into admissions at Baywood." Said Hutchison: "What appear to be community-minded efforts by the hospital to send guidance counselors, drug-abuse advisers, and other guest speakers into the public schools are motivated primarily by a desire to identify people who may be admitted to inpatient care."

Once, when occupancy rates in the hospital dropped to an "unacceptable level," Hutchison said he was ordered to move a number of patients from outpatient care into the hospital, with "no consideration shown to their clinical condition. The issue of whether or not anyone required inpatient care, from a medical standpoint, was not brought up."

The attitudes that Hutchison rebelled against seemed to be reflected in other facilities. In the summer of 1991, NME regional vice presidents and administrators, assembled for a national sales meeting, received a thick manual, marked "Confidential" that bore the title, "Inside Intake: Administrator Driven Intake Systems." The book offered a vast array of detailed suggestions to foster "an intake culture in the hospital"—that is, a system in which generating new admissions was paramount. "Make intake culture part of orientation for all new staff members," it advised.

The book was a blunt testament to the primacy of marketing, with clear instructions on setting monthly goals for converting various advertised "evaluation" programs—sessions designed to attract potential patients—into full-fledged "financially viable admissions." Administrators were exhorted to constantly monitor employee performance in converting inquiries into admissions.

Among the "expectations" the manual listed for the administrators to take back to their hospitals were that 70 percent to 80 percent of all telephone inquiries be scheduled for in-person evaluations, and 90 percent should take place within eighteen hours of the call. No-shows for appointments should be called "every thirty minutes" during an evaluating employee's shift, and afterward "a minimum of three more times on staggered shifts until contacted." Other suggestions given to the supervisors and administrators:

- Deal "pro-actively" with objections from physicians and nurses about bringing in "too many people" for evaluations.
- "Be vigilant against employees trying to help callers over the telephone instead of bringing them in for evaluation." Monitor incoming calls to ensure that "clinical screening" or "phone diagnosis" by "helpful" workers does not result in "lost admissions."
- Make "follow-up calls" to those who fail to show up for evaluation appointments, to ascertain "whether hospital staff created obstacles." For recalcitrant callers, paid taxi transportation to the hospital was suggested.
- At least half of those coming for evaluations should ultimately be admitted as patients. For those who demur, "Ask staff why

evaluations didn't convert." In tones that sounded more like they belonged on a used-car lot, the manual warned: "Admissions are lost when admissions don't occur the same day as the evaluation."

• Institute "monthly standards" for admissions employees and ensure that staff psychiatrists and nursing directors are aware that "inquiries and evaluations are their responsibility. Hold them accountable" and train medical staff to be "intake advocates" with "a sense of urgency to get admissions to happen."

• Be certain that business office managers understand "that insurance verification takes priority."

• Stress that courtesy counts in sales: "Communicate Thank-You" to referral sources who generate hospital admissions.

The manual also listed its "Golden Rules" for supervisors to teach admissions staff:

• When callers ask about the cost of hospital services, explain that "this will be addressed when they receive their evaluation." Callers should be reminded to bring their insurance cards.

• Let staff know that their "conversion rate"—the percentage of inquiries converted into admissions—is a crucial measure of individual job performance. Administrators should discuss an employee's conversion rate "openly" and "set monthly goals" for hospital admissions.

An NME manual entitled "Crisis Services," which was distributed to supervisors, administrators, and admissions staff in 1988, advised: "Hire a shark" to run hospital outreach crisis programs.

NME psychiatric hospitals also organized AMA ("Against Medical Advice") Teams, composed of doctors and other professionals, whose role was to dissuade patients from checking out early. NME marketing documents referred to community sources such as mental-health workers, school counselors, hospital room personnel, clergy people, corporate employee assistance program officials, police and probation officers as "gatekeepers," underscoring their potential for providing patients.

At corporate business gatherings, filling the beds in the psychiatric hospitals was always the major topic. In June 1989, at an annual marketing conference, program directors for NME psychiatric hospitals attended day-long workshops to share information about their successful promotional efforts. Here are some examples compiled from their reports:

• Los Altos Hospital in Long Beach, California, described its "Employee Answerline," a program in which forty-eight area companies, with a total of more than seven thousand employees, distributed a telephone number to call for help for emotional or substance abuse problems. The phone call went to the hospital, but the connection to a for-profit psychiatric hospital was kept in low profile. According to the report, "Operationally, the phone needs to be answered so the caller is not aware they are calling a hospital."

• Medfield Center in Largo, Florida, boasted of a program in which an average of five adolescents a month were admitted after attending informational sessions for "adolescents at risk." An estimated 90 percent of all admissions occurred at the time of consultation. Other "strong relationships" credited for yielding admissions were with schools and police departments that sponsored programs designed to divert youths arrested for minor infractions into treatment rather than jail. Medfield Center also reported that business and women's groups "have been great referral sources." One six-week promotion in the winter of 1988 cost $800 in expenses, chiefly for flyers, and yielded twelve female patients, all of whom had "commercial insurance."

Medfield also sought out "underachievers" among youths aged 10 to 17 with a promotion it called the Academic Motivation Program. It was launched with radio and print ads that defined underachievers as students whose performance in school was "substantially" below expectations and said, "Many studies indicate underachievers include as many as 50 percent of all school age children."

• Tidewater Psychiatric Hospital in Norfolk, Virginia, reported that its Student Assistance and Intervention Program (SAIP) was bringing in three to six admissions a month. Its theme was that as much as a third of any school's student population "is either involved in drugs or is considering suicide."

• Psychiatric Institute of Washington, D.C., said it racked up fifteen admissions from thirty evaluations in its ADVANCE program, described as "a psychoeducational program designed to access school gatekeepers" during summer vacation periods.

• The "Court Assistance Program" at Jefferson Hospital in Jefferson, Indiana, reported thirty-two admissions from forty-six evaluations referred by court and probation caseworkers. "Gatekeepers" were given promotional kits that included a bat, baseball cards, a cap, brochures, and a poster that said, "We Want to Play Ball." Attributing the success of the program to persistence by a marketing staff armed with a mailing list of court personnel, the hospital stressed: "The courts *must* feel that you are taking a burden from them."

• Laurelwood Hospital in Texas reported that one judge sent twenty-seven adolescents to its PALS (Prevention and Leadership School) program, "designed to develop referrals from probation departments and judges."

• Brawner Psychiatric Institute of Atlanta, Georgia, described success with its "You Deserve a BREAK" lunch. Invitations were sent to seventy-five local potential referral sources—doctors' office managers, secretaries, receptionists, and nurses—

for a free lunch program on dealing with difficult patients. Attendees went home with coffee mugs that featured the hospital's admissions number.

• Springwood Psychiatric Institute in Leesburg, Virginia, instituted a six-day inpatient treatment program for "adult children of dysfunctional families." The patients, all covered by insurance, were recruited from twelve-step groups like Alanon, or responded to advertisements that listed twelve characteristics of co-dependency, among them "an overdeveloped sense of responsiblity" to others and a need for "approval."

The hospital reported: "Co-dependency is popular with the media."

In 1990, at another NME annual conference, program directors and other staff members were exhorted to focus on the challenges and opportunities of "seasonal planning"—thinking ahead to try to keep beds occupied during Thanksgiving, Christmas, and summer vacation periods, when hospitals are traditionally less full and when some usual "referral sources," such as schools and EAPs, can't be fully tapped.

Though many of those attending were physicians, there was little talk of medicine. Instead, participants took part in sales conferences, pep rallies, inspirational group meetings, and even role-playing seminars in which the need to improve "patient census" was endlessly stressed. The PIA Marketeers heard tips on how to persuade patients thinking of discharging themselves (or their children) for the holidays—even for three-day holiday weekends—to stay around instead for the merry festivities. "Step up patient and family activities," said one tip listed in printed material for the conference. At Christmastime, for example, psychiatric hospitals could sponsor family parties and dinners, tree-trimming events on the children's ward, celebrity appearances, free family holiday photographs, gift-making classes, outings—anything to "prevent un-planned discharges."

In material for a role-playing session on "discharge intervention training," a fictitious scenario was offered to show how a patient's wish to take a Caribbean vacation might be turned aside. In the scenario, the husband of the patient makes an appeal to a nurse to have his wife released from the PIA hospital where she is being treated for depression, arguing that a vacation to the Bahamas will "cheer her up." The nurse responds that releasing the woman would be a bad idea, but that using the enticement of a future trip to the Bahamas would be a way to "motivate" her to complete her hospitalization "program goals."

Participants also were given material called a "Handling Objections Practice Sheet." Other material stressed that holidays were ideal times to hand-deliver gifts in order to cultivate community referral sources such as school counselors, emergency room workers, police officers, and crisis counselors.

In another sample role-playing scenario, a "PIA marketeer" is shown calling on a local psychologist and offering him help to lighten his workload over the Christmas season by fielding his crisis phone calls.

"Our Helpline is available around the clock during the holidays. You could instruct your answering service to have your clients call the Holiday Hotline in cases of crisis," the scenario has the marketing employee say. The material suggests employees point out that PIA also covers local universities' counseling centers in the same way during busy holiday periods when regular counselors are away.

In another session, an administrator bragged that he had his hospital relocate the admissions and information office, from the front lobby to farther inside the building—so prospective customers could not leave as easily.

•   •   •

Within the industry, NME was considered the best at infusing its hospital structures top to bottom with the marketing ethos. But the other chains were not sluggards. At Charter Hospital of Redlands, California, promotional material encouraged staff members to "take an active role in marketing our hospital" and in the process earn valuable points toward a week-long Caribbean cruise, called the "Cruise for Full" in honor of the goal of keeping the beds full. "Don't be left on the dock!!" the promotional brochure said. Generating an admission got the highest award, five points; points also were given for such accomplishments as "bringing a new or approved referral source" to the hospital for a lunch or tour.

In 1989 a Charter hospital in Las Vegas sent employees a nine-page marketing memo entitled "The Charter Challenge," which described a marketing program that "earns the employee bonus points that will result in cash, prizes and privileges." Extra bonus points were awarded to every employee whenever all of the hospital's eighty-four beds were full. The memo reminded employees of the importance of verifying potential patients' insurance coverage. "When there is any problem with an insurance . . . an insurance alert will be typed and distributed."

Charter hospitals in Nevada also ran newspaper ads geared toward enticing to their programs professional women, addicted gamblers, and those interested in learning how to "intervene" and compel a loved one to accept treatment.

All of these hospital programs were supervised by physicians, members of the psychiatric profession. Psychiatrists who worked for private psychiatric hospitals were considered to be integral to the marketing effort. In the company's 1981 annual report, John M. Stribling, a Charter executive responsible for developing new hospitals in North Carolina, approvingly cited the "cohesion between our medical and professional staffs."

As a rule, professional criticism came from outside psychiatry.

But even when they conceded that abuses in psychiatric hospitals constituted a major national scandal, many leading psychiatrists maintained publicly that the profession as a whole was blameless. In 1992, speaking on behalf of the Texas Society of Psychiatric Physicians, Deborah C. Peel, chief of psychiatry at an Austin general hospital, pointed out that "reprehensible" abuses flourish partly because the standards of admission for psychiatric hospitals are lower than those for general hospitals. "Recruiters are *not* advertising free workups, evaluations, or consultations for people with asthma, people with chest pain, people with high blood pressure, et cetera. They are not promising on billboards and television commercials to send outreach teams to people's homes to do free consultations."

By the nineties, Peel said, it was clear that psychiatric hospitals were paying "bounties to all sorts of people, including school counselors, clergy, policemen and admissions clerks, who recruited vulnerable, frightened, troubled people with real or fabricated mental illnesses or chemical dependency. We would all be very concerned if general hospitals were competing for patients in these ways, using methods blatantly designed to find and recruit patients who have good health insurance policies."

Dr. Peel blamed the problems on "nonphysicians." It was as if the psychiatrists were not in charge of the asylum after all.

CHAPTER TEN

....

MODERN WESTERN CONCEPTS OF MENTAL ILLNESS EMERGED
from the Middle Ages and in part reflected the established order's
alarm that people were starting to think for themselves. Forever
afterward, moralism, mysticism, pseudo-science, and politics have
battled for the soul of psychiatry.

Since it had the troops, in the form of jobs in public mental
institutions, politics usually prevailed, though it made accommo-
dations with the other forces. Psychiatry and government have
been closely aligned since the so-called Great Confinement of the
seventeenth and eighteenth centuries, when the insane were ware-
housed with the desititute, the incompetent, the crippled, the
senile, orphans, beggars, petty criminals, and other social outcasts.
Literally chained into such settings, subject to crude medical interventions such as bloodletting, those who weren't severely insane
in those places soon began acting that way. Self-perpetuating, the
practice of incarcerating the mentally ill, usually punitively, constantly justified itself in both moral and quasi-medical terms.

Psychiatry's first great reform came with a late-eighteenth-
century movement in France to abolish the "chains"—physical
restraints on mental patients—and replace them with a system of
humane treatment in which medical responsibility for the insane

171

was firmly established as a proper function of the rational state.

In the United States, there were just four public mental hospitals before 1830, housing only a few hundred patients. Most of the seriously mentally ill remained out of sight—at home with families, or in prisons. But as rapid industrialization tore at the social fabric, municipal and county authorities established workhouses and poorhouses to collect the growing numbers of people adjudged insane, and created a cadre of medically trained personnel—psychiatrists—to supervise them.

Psychiatrists always bristled at this custodial function, which carried low status along with the constant frustration involved in treating insanity, a seemingly incurable malady. For over a century, psychiatry has wrestled with the conflict presented by its ethical responsibilities toward the severely insane and its impulse to find a more congenial clientele outside of the asylums, where few patients were ever "cured."

The Civil War gave psychiatrists their first major opportunity to treat people not locked in asylums, providing them with access to a conscripted military force whose makeup more closely resembled that of society as a whole. At the same time, medical science was making revolutionary strides in isolating bacteria as causes of infectious diseases such as cholera. Anxious to don the cloak of science themselves, psychiatrists proposed that mental illness, too, had organic causes. Psychiatry soon began promoting itself as a full-fledged medical specialty, one responsible not only for treating mental illness but also for preventing its spread.

The profession's power, stemming largely from its affiliation with government, strenghtened considerably after the Civil War, as states built large centralized institutions to confine the mentally ill under humane medical supervision. Psychiatrists who administered these facilities had banded together in 1844 in a group called the Association of Medical Superintendents of American Institutions for the Insane. The group was renamed the American Medico-Psychological Association in 1882 to reflect psychiatry's growing claims of being a medical science and its disdain for its traditional custodial role. Today, the group, now called the American Psychiatric Association, is psychiatry's counterpart to the American Medical Association.

The profession's evolution is important because it helps to explain psychiatry's long-standing and unique ties to government—not only for funding, but for legal authority to intervene in society. Since its earliest days, psychiatry and government have shared mutual economic interests that often translated into political policy overlaid with a moral superstructure.

Besides providing custodial care for the insane, state asylums traditionally functioned as bureaucratic power centers rich with the currency of state politics: patronage jobs, which grew proportionally with the burgeoning numbers of patients. By 1904, state asylums housed 150,000 patients. At the start of the Second World War, there were 500,000 people in asylums. However, by that time, taxpayers had begun to balk at the immense costs of operating these institutions. In New York, for example, public mental-health services—primarily the asylums—accounted for a third of the state budget by the second half of the 1940s. So after the Second World War, when the federal government decided to become heavily involved in funding and setting policy for mental health, the states were only too happy to share the burden.

Meanwhile, psychiatry had again gone to war and come back with grand and expensive ideas. During the Second World War, psychiatrists in the military had been given sway not only to evaluate large populations outside the asylum, but also to implement theories about mental illness, organizational efficiency, and social adjustment. When the war ended, psychiatrists returned to civilian life enthusiastic about the potential to break their profession out of its own institutional chains and move it into the general population on a large scale, now with federal support. One of the leading voices for that initiative was a psychiatrist named Robert H. Felix, who would soon become the founding director of the National

173

Institute of Mental Health. Felix defined an ambitious new mission for psychiatry: fostering "the prevention of mental illness and the production of positive mental health" to ensure that "each citizen has optimum opportunities for sustained creative and responsible participation in the life of the community and for the development of his own particular potentialities." Psychiatrists, Felix insisted, had a responsibility to "go out and find the people who need help." As noted by E. Fuller Torrey in *Nowhere to Go*, a book on the depopulation of the state hospitals in the postwar era, Felix urged his colleagues to become involved with "education, social work, the churches, recreation, the courts," by way of fully integrating psychiatry into general society.

At the time, the federal government's role in civilian mental health was limited mostly to funding small research projects. But policy was rapidly changing. Shortly after the war ended, Major General Lewis B. Hershey, the autocratic director of the Selective Service System, testified before Congress that mental illness posed a previously unsuspected threat to America's hard-won national security and future domestic tranquility. Hershey said that of the 4.8 million men who received Army medical deferments during the war, more than 20 percent were rejected for psychiatric disorders. What's more, "mental diseases" accounted for a third of all wartime disability discharges, Hershey said. The psychiatric profession quickly echoed the alarm: Unless the federal government acted decisively, a mental-illness "epidemic" lay ahead for America.

Central to this drive was the theory that psychiatry, no less than other medical fields such as immunology, offered a "preventive" therapeutic model that could identify mental illness early and alleviate its spread. At the same time, public attitudes toward the treatment of the severely mentally ill were changing because of exposés of deplorable conditions in state hospitals. First came a spate of widely publicized reports on abuses, issued by conscientious objectors who had spent the war years working in institutions.

Then came two influential books: In 1946, *The Snake Pit*, a best-selling novel by Mary Jane Ward, depicted the horrifying experiences of a "happily married" woman, "broken by the strains of modern living," who is committed to a state mental hospital. Two years later, a heavily illustrated book, *The Shame of the States* by Albert Deutsch, exposed the squalor and abject wretchedness of mental-hospital life.

The federal floodgates opened, pouring out money to train new mental-health professionals. This largesse revolutionized mental-health policy and subsidized a spectacular growth in psychiatry as well as in related professions such as psychology and psychiatric social work. Over the next thirty years, federal grants for the training of psychiatrists alone would exceed $2 billion. However, although it was partly spurred by demands for reforms in treating the severely insane, the federal effort was overwhelmingly directed toward mental-health work within the general population. In 1946, there were approximately three thousand psychiatrists in the United States; about two thirds of them worked in state mental hospitals. By 1956, there were about ten thousand psychiatrists—but only 17 percent now worked in public hospitals. In 1985, long after state mental hospitals had been virtually emptied by the movement known as deinstitutionalization, there were more than 32,000 psychiatrists. Most of them were now affiliated with revenue-generating hospitals.

In the fifties came another important milestone: The pharmaceutical industry began introducing a long line of psychiatric medications, such as Thorazine, which was hailed as a miracle drug that, with proper community supervision, enabled people to live outside asylums. These pharmaceutical advances helped to accelerate the emptying of state hospitals—which had 552,000 patients in 1955, and only 116,000 by 1984—and also to establish psychiatry more firmly in the ranks of biological medicine. Though psychiatrists trained in Freudian and other psychoanalytical theories still had considerable influence, especially in private practices with

175

wealthy clienteles in older urban areas, these therapists were rapidly becoming the old guard. The new breed of scientifically oriented psychiatrists pouring out of medical schools were disciples
of the theory that psychiatric disorders are biological diseases of
the brain, treatable by drugs in medical settings such as hospitals,
not by time-consuming talk and interminable counseling.

The needs of the seriously mentally ill—a population increasingly
adrift on the streets of American cities as asylums shut down—
went largely unmet. In the early 1960s, President Kennedy called
for a national mental-health policy that "relies primarily upon the
new knowledge and new drugs . . . which make it possible for most
of the mentally ill to be successfully and quickly treated in their
own communities." It was a policy that would enlist not only medical professionals, but also schools, social workers, and crisis counselors in an effort to provide comprehensive treatment in a national
network of two thousand community mental-health centers.

During the Johnson administration, Congress enthusiastically
made money available for this new era of mental health. In 1963,
total government spending on public mental health was about a
billion dollars a year—about 96 percent of which was still provided
by individual states. Within three years, the sum had jumped to
more than $17 billion, now overwhelmingly coming from the fed-
eral government.

Yet as the money flowed, treating the seriously mentally ill became secondary to the more agreeable task of promoting mental
health among the well. About six hundred community mental-
health centers did open, but few of them provided acute inpatient
care and emergency treatment, which are the services most needed
by seriously mentally ill people outside an insititution. In a 1966
report on the broken promise of community mental-health centers,
psychologists M. Brewster Smith and Nicholas Hobbs lamented
that "most of our therapeutic talent, often trained at public expense,
has been invested in solving not our hard-core mental-health problem—the psychotic of marginal competence and social status—but

in treating the relatively well-to-do educated neurotic." The community centers didn't even call patients "patients" anymore, E. Fuller Torrey noted. Instead, they became " 'clients' . . . individuals with problems of living—the teenaged son who refused to do what his parents told him, the wife whose husband was hinting at divorce, the man whose midlife crisis had made him depressed."

By the 1980s, with private health-insurance money flooding into the high end of the mental-health and addiction-treatment field, the record of deinstitutionalization was abundantly clear. In a 1981 editorial, *The New York Times* called the policy "a cruel embarrassment, a reform gone terribly wrong." The evidence of that failure was all around. "Not since the 1820s have so many mentally ill individuals lived untreated in public shelters, on the streets and in jails," said a report commissioned in 1990 by the Public Citizen Health Research Group and the National Alliance for the Mentally Ill. The report declared that the largest "de facto mental hospital in the U.S. is the Los Angeles County jail, where there are 3,600 inmates who are seriously mentally ill on an average day," seven hundred more than were in the nation's largest mental hospital. Charging that psychiatry had abadoned the severely mentally ill for lucrative private practices or the lure of investor-owned hospitals, the report concluded that there had been a "near total breakdown in public psychiatric services in the United States."

CHAPTER ELEVEN

....

SINCE RELATIVELY FEW USE IT, MOST PEOPLE STILL THINK OF psychiatry as a practice conducted in a private office, with a physician taking notes and a patient reposing on a couch or a comfortable stuffed chair, talking through his or her problems. But except for enclaves of urban affluence, where people can afford to pay for the attention, such private practices are becoming a thing of the past. Psychiatry is now a profession mostly focused on the corporate hospital rather than the private office.

In 1989, office visits to psychiatrists accounted for a mere 2.4 percent of the total 692 million office visits to physicians, while the profession itself has grown robustly. Virtually all of the growth has been in treating new diagnoses of illnesses and disorders once considered mere personal problems—spurred by the willingness of insurers to pay for treating them, usually with reimbursement policies tied, as they are in general medical care, to hospital procedures.

In 1986 (the last year in which federal statistics were kept for such classifications), 49 percent of inpatient admissions to private psychiatric hospitals were for diagnoses under the classification of "affective disorders" (later renamed mood disorders), a diagnostic term that defines various behaviors associated with mild to severe ranges of depression and changes in mood, including "manic episode" ("Frequently the person does not recognize that he or she is ill," according to the psychiatry's official clinical definition of the disorder). The same year, by comparison, such diagnoses represented 16.5 percent of the admissions to state and county mental hospitals, where the chronically mentally ill are most often housed.

With the triumph of "biopsychiatry," and the rise of its practitioners as significant revenue producers in the hospital industry, the days of toiling for the government in the snake pits have become merely grim historical references to most psychiatrists.

In hospitals, "psychiatrists were viewed until fairly recently as one step above stargazers," said Ira Schwartz, the Michigan youth-policy researcher. Beholden to a range of diagnoses largely confined to the seriously mentally ill (who tend to be poor), "they were not able to generate the billings; they had low professional status in hierarchy." But in the eighties, "all of a sudden, the psychiatrists started to gain respect among their colleagues in hospitals," Schwartz said.

By and large, psychiatry has succeeded in establishing itself as a component of medical science, despite the warnings of in-house critics such as Peter Breggin, the psychiatrist who has written about the dangers of modern organized psychiatry, which he dismisses as a "mishmash of philosophy, psychology, religion, law enforcement and politics, as well as social engineering and big business, and occasionally science and medicine."

Whether bible or textbook, the American Psychiatric Association's *Diagnostic and Statistical Manual of Mental Disorders, Third Edition, Revised (DSM-III-R)*, a glossary of disorders and behaviors that the psychiatric establishment categorizes as mental illnesses, is the clinical basis for today's psychiatry.

DSM-III-R was published in 1987, but a year later the American Psychiatric Association began preparing a new edition, *DSM-IV*, which is eagerly anticipated by biopsychiatrists for its anticipated deemphasis of anecdotal evidence and opinion in favor of the kinds of clinical documentation (including laboratory and field tests) that imply scientific credibility and conform more readily to insurance reimbursement criteria. *DSM-IV*, according to an article in the *American Journal of Psychiatry*, will finally succeed in erasing the "unfortunate" distinction that still exists in the lay world between mental disorder and physical disease.

The new *DSM* is also expected to greatly expand the range of diagnoses for child and adolescent problems, such as "oppositional defiant disorder," as well as disorders exclusive to women, and to present clinical evidence to establish such problems as sleep disorders, binge eating, and seasonal affective disorders as mental illnesses. As organized psychiatry expands globally—and as U.S. corporate psychiatric hospitals open facilities abroad, chiefly in Western Europe—*DSM-IV* also will strive to become more compatible with the International Classification of Diseases codes in wide use throughout world medicine.

Even as it is being rewritten, the existing *DSM* stands as a neological masterwork. For clinicians, researchers and patients, it defines a language to label as mental diseases a vast range of common and uncommon behaviors, from "severe psychosis" to "self-defeating personality disorder" to "nicotine dependence"; at all stages of life, from "reactive attachment disorder of infancy" to "senile dementia," providing clinical legitimacy for claims about what the psychiatric journals now routinely call "the rising pandemic of mental disorders."

With its detailed index of hundreds of cross-referenced symptoms, *DSM-III-R* is a long way from the earliest Western classifications of mental illness, which sprang from ancient Greece, where Hippocrates posited four temperaments: choleric, sanguine, melancholic, and phlegmatic.

In 1840, the U.S. census listed only a single harsh category of mental disorder, "idiocy," though even this constituted a great advance from the earliest days of modern psychiatry, in the sev-

181

enteenth century, when Satan was considered one of the primary causes of insanity, especially among women.

The modern American psychiatric propensity for classifying mental illnesses in exhaustive detail owes much to Benjamin Rush, a signer of the Declaration of Independence and the chief physician of the Continental Army. Rush is considered the father of American psychiatry; his image adorns the official seal of the American Psychiatric Association. Sociologist Phil Brown, writing in the *Journal of Mind and Behavior* in 1990, noted that among Rush's contributions to psychiatric nosology—classification of diseases—was "anarchia," defined as a brain disease of people who were unhappy with the new American political system. Rush was also one of the first to declare that drunkenness was a mental illness.

Over the years, definitions of mental disorders expanded to meet social and political concerns at least as much as medical ones. Before the Civil War, psychiatrists in the South added their own unique contributions, discovering, for example, a mental illness called drapetomania. This disorder occurred only in black slaves and was characterized by a desire to run away.

Refined, expanded, contrived, even discarded when political winds changed direction, classifications of mental illness entered this century designed chiefly to facilitate statistical tabulation in the bureaucracy of mental asylums. But after the Second World War, as federal money poured into mental health, psychiatry moved more confidently into concern about the neuroses, personality disorders, and anxieties of the general population. In a field dominated by subjective assessments, government financing and supervision helped induce pressure for a common reference. In 1952, the first *Diagnostic and Statistical Manual of Mental Disorders (DSM-I)*, heavily influenced by psychotherapy, codified American psychiatry's nomenclature for mental illness.

By the time *DSM-II* arrived in 1968, as federal policies and funding requirements aided the cause of biomedical approaches to mental illness, psychiatry was well on its way back to its pre-

Freudian roots in clinical disease concepts. Deemphasizing the role of social environment in favor of more easily quantifiable biological data, *DSM-II* and its successors were increasingly influenced by the pharmaceutical industry, whose widely acclaimed "miracle drugs," liberating the insane asylums, had spawned second- and third-generation tranquilizers and antidepressants that psychiatrists were disseminating into the general population.

More recent *DSM* innovations, much welcomed by the now-dominant investor-owned and profit-driven psychiatric industry, included classifications of multiple diagnoses (alcoholism in tandem with depression, for example). More intricate classifications for children and adolescents also evolved, thanks to the influence of the rapidly growing ranks of child psychiatrists and psychologists. The growth in labels was impressive. In 1952, the first *DSM* listed sixty classifications of mental illness. *DSM-II* had more than twice that. With the publication of *DSM-III* in 1980, there were more than two hundred. *DSM-IV* will add still more.

Inexorably, as psychiatry refocused itself on the disease model, it promulgated the theory that mental illness is basically a brain disease. In 1989, President Bush designated the 1990s the "Decade of the Brain," marking the triumph of biopsychiatry, which had by then forged links with the leading U.S. medical schools.

On January 1, 1990, California became the first state to declare officially that certain mental illnesses are actually biologically based brain diseases, caused by malfunctions and malformations of the brain. This was more than a nod to psychiatry's most important modern dogma. The California law, strenuously lobbied for by psychiatrists and psychiatric hospitals, mandated that employer insurance benefits cover "schizophrenia, schizo-affective disorders, bipolar and delusional depressions and pervasion development disorder" in the same way as they covered physical diseases.

It had been an uphill fight for biopsychiatrists, who had languished for years in the professional shadow of older, analytically trained psychiatrists, who tended to have the most influential connections and the best-established private practices. In 1970, twenty-five years after federal funding began subsidizing the training of large numbers of psychiatrists, the profession still hadn't found a profitable role within the general population. There were too many psychiatrists, too few jobs in hospitals, and not enough patients willing or able to pay the kinds of fees a doctor needed to charge to devote an hour exclusively to listening to someone's problems. Young psychiatrists were acutely aware of the fabulous amounts of money being made by their classmates from medical school who had gone into other specialties, such as cardiology or orthopedics, where they were able to see several patients an hour *and* share in the even bigger profits available from insurance payments for attending many of those patients in a hospital.

Along with the tenfold increase in the ranks of psychiatrists from 1945 to 1985 there had been a corresponding jump in the number of other professionals in mental-health care. Over the same period, the ranks of psychologists also increased tenfold, to about 45,000, and psychiatric social workers' ranks increased 27-fold, to more than 54,000, according to E. Fuller Torrey's *Nowhere to Go*. With large numbers of nonphysician psychotherapists and counselors hanging out shingles and offering similar services at lower costs, psychiatrists who depended on talk therapy were becoming an endangered species, restricted largely to clients in affluent urban areas—to people who, almost by definition, were seldom impaired enough to require medical treatment under existing guidelines for mental illness. For psychiatrists, things looked glum.

Throughout the 1970s, with state hospitals emptying out, psychiatry's existence as a viable medical specialty was threatened. By 1980, the proportion of graduating medical students selecting psychiatric residencies had dropped to a record low of 2.6 percent (down from an average of over 10 percent in the 1950s and 1960s). What's more, with hospitals spending millions on the latest technological diagnostic marvels, it was the Triumph of Science—doctors were the kids who had excelled in chemistry class, not in philosophy or psychology. (By 1989, only 4 percent of U.S. medical students would have liberal-arts degrees.) To most eager young physicians, private-practice psychiatry, characterized by extended sessions of listening to people go on about personal and highly subjective experiences, seemed ludicrously out-of-date.

Psychiatry became fully "remedicalized" amid massive marketing by both hospitals and drug companies and a great rush into medical schools, occasioned by the gold strike of federal Medicare and Medicaid funds. From 1955 to 1975, the number of people entering medical schools nearly doubled. By the seventies, with insurance money starting to flow and encouraging new private psychiatric hospitals to sprout all over the country, psychiatric residencies suddenly began to pick up. With new opportunities beckoning, the ranks of first-year residents in psychiatry shot up 40 percent during the eighties, accelerating in the last half of the decade, during the peak of expansion for private psychiatric hospitals, and falling off again once that business slowed in the nineties.

The American Psychiatric Association, long battered by internal conflicts over the direction of psychiatry, had meanwhile found its own white knight in the pharmaceutical industry. In the mid-1980s, drug companies were contributing at least 20 percent of the group's revenue. "By 1987, the APA annual meeting had become a drug company circus," Peter Breggin wrote in *Toxic Psychiatry*. At the 1992 APA meeting, drug manufacturers sponsored dozens of symposia over five days, on subjects such as "The Elderly: Today's Treatment Challenge," and "Therapeutic Strategies for the Patient With Treatment Resistant Anxiety." Drug companies are also by far the leading funding sources for academic research in psychiatry today.

"Psychiatrists and drug companies both benefit from their intercourse—the first because the image of doctors prescribing medicines to treat mental illnesses bolsters the medical model, the second because their medicines sell," Dr. Ronald Leifer wrote in 1990 in the *Journal of Mind and Behavior*.

The influence of the drug industry, pervasive at all levels of modern psychiatry, even challenges the axiom that there is no such thing as a free lunch. For example, at a leading center for training psychiatrists, Columbia Presbyterian Medical Center in New York, drug-company sales representatives regularly provide free lunches for residents, who are regaled with promotions for psychiatric drugs.

By the end of the eighties, millions of Americans who had never before come into contact with psychiatry were using greatly expanded health-insurance benefits and spending stretches of time in the new psychiatric hospitals—twenty to thirty days, on average, rather than the five or six days a patient with a serious medical problem might spend in a general hospital. It was the triumph of medically oriented psychiatry, a profession which, according to Breggin, exists now at "the political center of a multi-billion-dollar psycho-pharmaceutical complex that pushes biological and genetic theories, as well as drugs, on the society. It is a political institution licensed by the state, financed by government, and empowered by the courts."

For a new generation of psychiatrists, the best jobs now were in the new corporate hospitals, which aggressively recruited psychiatrists, whose signatures are needed to admit patients and prescribe drugs. While most believed in their ethical independence as physicians, the system they entered was not designed to brook resistance that got in the way of profits.

"It's not really well known that psychiatrists lost control of psychiatric hospitals five or ten years ago," said Agnes Whitley, a psychiatrist who quit one private psychiatric hospital in disgust in 1983.

To the corporate hospitals, the most highly valued psychiatrists were those with established outside practices that could be used as pipelines for patient admissions. All over the country, corporate psychiatric hospitals operate programs to maintain the goodwill of and get referrals from regional physicians—psychiatrists and medical specialists alike. An example was NME's Kingwood Hospital in Michigan City, Indiana, not far from Chicago, which set up its "Physician's Ambassador Program" in 1988. Kingwood's sales brochure, distributed to area psychiatrists, stated: "Kingwood's Ambassadors can help you define an effective marketing approach specific to your specialty area. We'll ensure you media exposure."

But even those without private practices were avidly sought. A highly respected psychiatrist who had set up community health programs in New York State recalled his first encounters with the corporate psychiatric industry:

"Around 1985, they started heavily recruiting state psychiatrists. The pitch was persuasive for someone being ground down by the frustrations of dealing with the mental-health bureaucracy, which by then had become the Siberia of state government. Conditions were pitiful—every day Albany was pulling the rug out from under me. So these private guys had a pretty good pitch when you first met them. It was 'Hey, Doc, wouldn't you rather be dealing with nice, affluent patients who had some motivation behind them? Wouldn't you like an easier practice?' They were talking lots of money, too—not just salaries, but facilities, staff. Some days, after dealing with what I had to deal with, I'd come home bushwhacked and just stare at those offers.

"For a psychiatrist who wasn't too troubled by his conscience, it could be an easy life," this doctor said. But "you heard that the psychiatrists who had gone to work for them in other states were under heavy pressure in terms of diagnosis."

The dilemma underscored the major issue confronting psychiatry today: the ethics of providing mental-health care in an atmosphere of profit incentives.

"The hucksters moved in and swept a good number of young psychiatrists into their programs," said Frank P. Schuster, a former president of the Texas Society of Psychiatric Physicians. "The lure was bucks, lots of bucks—six figures, right out of their residency training." From the start, Schuster said, the hospitals' goal was clear: "Keep patients the maximum time that their insurance covered them."

Dr. Victor Weiss, a former medical director at a private psychiatric hospital in San Antonio, said that a San Angelo psychiatric hospital once offered him $1,500 for every patient he brought in.

"I said 'Wow, I don't take bribes,' " Weiss recalled.

Another psychiatrist who resisted the blandishments was Charles S. Arnold of San Antonio, who recalled being approached in June 1984 by an executive from a corporate-owned psychiatric hospital. Arnold, who had already heard rumors about the hospital's aggressive tactics for generating business, was so suspicious that he surreptitiously tape-recorded the interview, which took place in his office.

After a preliminary explanation of how psychiatrists were becoming rich working for private hospitals, the interviewer got right to the point, sounding out Dr. Arnold's willingness to tailor a diagnosis for payment: "Where are your loyalties?" the corporate recruiter asked rhetorically. "I mean, if we're going to give you a patient and make you fifteen thousand dollars just for not having to do a damn thing but write your name and admit him, or if I've got a patient for you to admit—if I put him there and I give you that patient, why not give us the [psychological] testing? If I say, 'Dr. Arnold, I've got a patient that I want admitted under major depression,' will you admit him?"

The overture was not subtle, Arnold said. "It was rephrased over and over again: 'If you will simply go along with the program and change your way of thinking, we will do your work for you. All you have to do is drop by [the hospital] and say hello, and you can bill the insurance company for a hundred, a hundred twenty-five dollars a day [for each patient].' "

The money available for signing on with the private hospital sounded staggering. "I have specific knowledge of at least one case where a psychiatrist had thirty-five patients in the hospital—and nobody in the world can take care of that many people—charging

[each] a hundred dollars a day. That's in the neighborhood of ninety thousand to a hundred thousand dollars a month!" Dr. Arnold said.

A plentiful supply of patients would be easier to ensure once he worked for the hospital, Dr. Arnold was told.

The interviewer recounted how another psychiatrist had been recruited with this approach: "Look, you want to be rich? You let us set up this program the way we want to set it up, all you do is be the admitting psychiatrist, and we'll make you rich."

Arnold was so bothered by what he had heard that he called his lawyer and wrote the U.S. Department of Health and Human Services a letter reporting the experience. He cited a combination of factors for what had gone wrong with corporate psychiatry. Among them: The American Psychiatric Association's expanding *DSM* classifications of "illnesses or disorders, many of which are not actually illnesses" but are designed to create a demand for treatment and pressure for insurance coverage; heavy advertising and promotion; the "programmatic" concept of treatment characterized by all-encompassing "milieu" therapy; the diminishment of the doctor-patient relationship as private psychiatry withered; and "the application of psychiatry to resolve many situations that are actually social problems."

Dr. Arnold identified the hospital that approached him as Park North Hospital, which was later sold and renamed Colonial Hills— the hospital where Jeramy Harrell was held.

Arnold said he was not left with any illusions about the nobility of his profession. While many psychiatrists and other mental-health professionals resisted offensive inducements, a dismaying number "betrayed the public trust and in effect sold their souls," he said. "Sure, there are a large number of honest and ethical psychiatric and mental-health-care providers. However, the number that are motivated by greed rather than concern for the health of the patient—or by sound scientific, ethical practice—is alarmingly high."

Some psychiatrists signed on with psychiatric hospitals and eventually walked out in disgust. A Texas psychiatrist who ran adolescent programs at Charter Hospital in Grapevine and Green Oaks Hospital in Dallas told the *Dallas News* in 1991 that he quit after he began thinking of himself as a "medical slave." The psychiatrist, Dr. James Grubbs, added, "My basic strategy for dealing with the pressures that the for-profit hospitals are brought under is to not work there, to vote with my feet."

Here and there, other psychiatrists went public (when they could get someone to listen) to describe what some of them feared were systemic abuses both in free-standing corporate hospitals and in psychiatric programs of for-profit general hospitals. Among them were: diagnoses being crossed out overnight, with new ones better suited to insurance benefits substituted; drugs administered, without the attending physician's approval, by young psychiatrists recruited fresh out of medical school; incessant pressure to meet quotas, with physicians evaluated on the basis of how long their patients remained in the hospital; pressure to move patients who had exhausted benefits in one category of mental disorder to a new category with benefits remaining.

Kenneth M. Clark, a Nevada psychiatrist, told investigators in 1992 about a CHAMPUS patient in an HCA psychiatric facility in Reno, whose benefits had run out, "at which point the hospital shifted the billing from the patient's name to his brother's name, even though the brother never was and never had been hospitalized."

Writing in the *Medical Tribune* in 1987 one jaded psychiatrist said of corporate psychiatry:

> *Diagnosis, surely, is important as a psychiatric function. Not really. There must be a diagnosis on the chart, but scientific rigor and correctness are less important than "sensitivity to the reimbursement implications." . . . Yet for-profit psychiatric hospitals do not lack for psychiatrists. The lure they offer is "easy money," of course. Their marketing efforts, we are told, will expand the pie by luring people into treatment who oth-*

*erwise would never see a psychiatrist, and thus feed patients
to an affiliated psychiatrist. . . . And then there is the offer of
a retainer to be a "medical director" of something or other. . . .
Rarely does the psychiatrist have any authority to direct anything or anyone; and if he naively does try to direct, he is quickly
reminded by the corporate boss who is really in charge. . . .
And then there is the inexorable pressure to fill beds. If in doubt,
admit. The "best" psychiatrist, in the eyes of the corporation,
is the one who admits a very high percentage of his new patients
for inpatient treatment. [However,] professional norms recognize that the best psychiatrist is often the one who admits the
smallest percentage of his patients for inpatient treatment."*

The disgruntled psychiatrist closed with advice to his colleagues:

*Take nothing from the corporation until you have determined
unequivocally, without any wishful thinking, what you are giving in return (for there will be a quid pro quo, you can count
on it.) . . . Do not for a moment believe that loyalty or other
sentimental issues will influence your longevity with the company in the least; when you no longer are of sufficient value as
an exploitable resource, you will be jettisoned. Keep your suitcase packed!*

Implicit, if unspoken, in many arrangements between hospitals and
psychiatrists was the importance the corporation placed on maintaining "patient census"—keeping the beds full of paying customers. Some arrangements were more specific.

At Belmont Hills Hospital, a facility owned by Community Psychiatric Centers, in Belmont, California, an employment contract
renewal offered in 1989 to the psychiatrist who was director of the
adolescent program stipulated that 15 of the 18 beds in the adolescent unit needed to be occupied and that "stagnation" in patient

levels was a serious concern. "We need your involvement to more actively market" the adolescent program, the contract stated.

When the contract offered to the Belmont Hills physician became public, CPC president Loren B. Shook denied that the language constituted a quota that the doctor was expected to meet, and described it instead as a general guideline about the program's goals.

The contract also emphasized the importance of maintaining a "dual diagnosis" attitude in admissions. Dual diagnoses are one of the most profitable trends in corporate psychiatry, offering opportunities to obtain insurance reimbursement for a second disorder once the benefits on the first have expired. The concept was described in a 1990 ad by another institution, Gracie Square Hospital in New York, which stated that problems such as substance abuse are often accompanied by other related mental disorders, and advised: "It often doesn't work to treat one without the other. . . ."

CHAPTER TWELVE

....

"THE ONE THING THAT JUST TERRORIZED THOSE PEOPLE WAS that some poor son of a bitch like me could just walk in the door and stumble onto what they were doing," Bill Coakley said with a small, weary chuckle. "All I wanted to do was solve the problem, nothing else. They absolutely could not figure out what my game was."

Coakley was reminiscing about his unexpected six-month career detour in 1986 and 1987 as a tormentor of psychiatric hospitals in the vicinity of West Palm Beach, Florida.

Coakley and his friend, Debbie Wescott, live together in a small but airy garden apartment in Lantana, a middle-class island in the affluent archipelago of the Gold Coast of south Florida, tucked behind the front range of condominiums facing the sea.

They are a pleasant couple, even-tempered, quietly affectionate, as hospitable to a visitor as they are to the daily effusion of wild birds—blue jays, grackles, the occasional cardinal and wood-pecker—who alight on the windowsill, sometimes hopping over to the counter or the desk to snatch a peanut left out in a bowl.

In his early forties, Coakley composes, teaches college courses in music technology, and installs sound systems for a living; a decade younger, Debbie works as a secretary. Seen together, they seem still in bloom from a more conscientious era—the late sixties, perhaps. It is not surprising to learn that they spent a good amount of time together brandishing picket signs, once Bill got into his crusade and wouldn't let go.

The institution that first got his attention was Lake Hospital, one of several psychiatric hospitals in the region owned by NME. Actually, Coakley's association with Lake Hospital had started out amicably enough: He was hired to design a public-relations campaign for it, a project he that took on with enthusiasm early in 1986 before he blew the job by blowing the whistle.

Today, as the psychiatric-hospital industry wonders about the trouble it has recently seen, a look back at people like Coakley and Wescott provides a small lesson in the ability of ordinary citizens to expose wrongdoing, once they get their dander up.

"I didn't have any ax to grind," Coakley says today of his experience. To the contrary, Coakley had approached the psychiatric business quite approvingly, fully prepared to sing its praises. That was late in 1985, when he became interested in addiction-treatment programs after he helped a friend whose daughter had hit bottom with a severe drug problem. The friend had borrowed $5,000 to admit the teenage girl to a for-profit addiction center—not a full-fledged psychiatric hospital of the sort being opened all over the region, but a smaller drug-addiction and alcoholism treatment facility housed in a rambling cottage beside the ocean.

To lend support, Coakley accompanied his friend to several group sessions while the girl was undergoing treatment. Although he was favorably impressed with the films shown and with the words spoken about addiction, he found himself, in an idle moment, gazing at the faces of the assembled young addicts, all of them chastened, all apparently motivated to recover—and all of them, he mused, having paid $5,000 for a two-week program.

"I was looking at these fourteen patients, thinking: 'Fourteen times five thousand dollars—hey, that's not too shabby.' Mentally, I worked through the money, trying to see how much could you spend on maintenance in this place; how much for food, mortgage, salaries—the staff seemed to be all former addicts or low-paid counselors; a secretary, maybe a groundskeeper or maintenance man of some kind. I thought: '*I can't begin to spend the money.*' "

When Thanksgiving approached, his friend said she had to come up with more money to keep her daughter in over the holiday. The girl herself explained to him, "They said I'm not ready to go yet. It looks like I'm going to be here for another three or four weeks."

"Whatever it takes," he replied gently, although he actually couldn't see a good reason to keep her there.

"Well, there's not many other people here," the girl said sadly, her face showing a fear of abandonment.

Not long after, Coakley understood. The facility had applied pressure to keep her there, so that revenue would flow during the slack holiday period. This insight occurred to Coakley much later after he began looking into the private psychiatric hospital industry.

In 1986, Lake Hospital commissioned Coakley to put together a promotional presentation, "a facelift," he said, designed around "a video to give them a new image and augment their advertising. They wanted to use it for special presentations to Lions Clubs and other community groups—a 'We care' kind of thing, 'We're here to help the community.' "

Coakley's friend, Wescott, remembered: "At first I didn't think anything of it—just another slide-presentation job. But then he got hold of the information that showed him how much they were charging, and he was coming home like, 'This is incredible! Look at these prices!' and I knew we were in for an adventure."

In putting the presentation together, Coakley interviewed many hospital staff members and had free run of the facility. Glowing tributes to the quality of care flowed, dutifully recorded. Coakley had to work hard to show the hospital's physical plant at its best; the truth was, it wasn't much to look at. The building had once been Lake Worth General Hospital, which NME had purchased and renovated, but the result was "a barrackslike affair," he said. Still, "the presentation was coming together famously. They were going to love it."

Until the day a nurse snorted derisively when Coakley told her how impressed he was with the hospital's good work. Intrigued, he drew her aside for a quiet talk. At the end of their enlightening discussion, she slipped him a confidential hospital notebook that listed, in great detail, how much patients' insurance companies were being charged, and for what.

"What a shot in my balloon!" he said. He kept looking at the list of charges, saying "The decimal points can't be in the right place." He looked again at the rundown facilities and the low-paid staff. He began nosing around.

"I guess you stay in pretty close contact with these people after they leave the hospital?" he asked one head nurse in a ward.

"For what?" she replied.

There was no aftercare; Coakley could discern little interest in how patients fared once they left. There was exceedingly high interest, however, in insurance coverage. Furthermore, while Alcoholics Anonymous and other cost-free groups were allowed to use a hospital meeting room, the benevolence seemed to have a purpose: insurance evaluation and recruiting of potential patients.

In the adolescent classroom, he noticed peeling paint, exposed ductwork, electrical-wire conduit nailed to the walls, "a four-foot-long chalkboard that you would normally find in a child's bedroom." And, he ascertained, the teachers were paid by the local school district, not the hospital.

Elsewhere, Coakley counted as many as twenty patients packed to a unit with two small bathrooms that would have been at home in a badly managed gas station. He took in little things like cheap curtains, big things like old, broken, rusty exercise equipment that looked as if it had been donated by the Salvation Army. Again, he referred to the book that listed all the charges. *Recreational therapy?*

"The place is a rat hole," he told Wescott. "What . . . a . . . *ripoff*." Characteristically, he ran the numbers: "What have they got invested here? An old building with beds, makeshift wards, cheap plumbing, an X-ray machine like you'd find in any chiropractor's office."

Meanwhile, the local airwaves were full of advertising claims for psychiatric hospitals, which were sprouting like fast-food joints on a new stretch of highway. In Palm Beach County, the number of private psychiatric hospitals went from three to ten *in two years*, from 1985 to 1987. The money was flowing. In 1986, Blue Cross/ Blue Shield of Florida payments for psychiatric and substance-abuse treatment increased more than three times faster than those for all other areas of health care.

Looking beyond Lake Hospital, Coakley was amazed at the claims being made on the airwaves and in printed ads, which he described as: "Does your teenager hate to come home to dinner? Does he sulk around? All a simple phone call away for help." Another ad he recalled as: "Thirty-four questions to see if your child is hyperactive—Does your child rush through his schoolwork without checking it over? . . .Do you or your spouse have to keep after your child to do his chores? . . .Does your child seem to wear out clothes and toys too quickly?" . . . If the answer was yes to "more than a few" of the questions, it was time to look for help. Coakley muttered, "This is something you put a kid in a mental hospital for?"

Once Coakley got fired up, investigating the psychiatric business became virtually a full-time preoccupation. He discovered "interlocking networks for referrals . . . involving even the nonprofit mental-health facilities in the area," which were rewarded for cooperation with the occasional free bed for a charity case—"all skewed to funneling insurance money into the corporate hospitals."

Before long, Coakley and Wescott were showing up at shopping centers with stacks of fliers that listed price comparisons and pointed out that drug treatment for those unable to pay was increasingly unavailable, while even for those who could pay, it made sense to shop around, even if the insurance company was footing the bill. Coakley said: "For less than $1,500 a patient can get essentially the same addiction-treatment program" that private psychiatric hospitals were charging ten times more for.

Coakley devoted a good six months to his campaign while Wescott took on a second job to pay the bills. Why? "He wanted to see if one person could make a difference," she said simply, as if that was answer enough.

Unluckily for the hospitals, Coakley liked to talk and came across well on television and radio. In November 1986, he was interviewed on the local public broadcasting station and delivered a detailed critique of the private hospitals' "enormous public-relations campaign" to exploit addiction and emotional distress.

In interviews, Coakley began denouncing the well-publicized Fair Oaks 800-COCAINE hot line. He and Wescott did an informal survey, interviewing twenty people at random to ask what they knew about the hot line. "Eighteen of them thought it was a government agency," he said. None knew that the hot line went directly into an office at Fair Oaks Hospital in Delray Beach—a hospital that operated, Coakley discovered through detailed cost comparisons, the most expensive alcohol- and drug-abuse program in Florida.

Finally, he became a regular guest of Don Silverman, who had a popular local talk radio program on WJNO-AM.

Coakley's lack of a hidden agenda impressed him. "I can't find the gimmick," Silverman told his listeners, many of whom responded with their own complaints about private psychiatric hospitals, often involving adolescent care. These included the case of a teenage girl who had spent fifteen weeks at Fair Oaks in 1987, after her mother saw the hospital's ads for treating teenage "behavior problems." The total hospital bill was $82,000. Or the complaint of another mother that her daughter returned from twelve weeks (and $50,000 worth) of drug-abuse treatment at Lake Hospital under heavy medication that itself had become addicting. "It was like talking to a seashell," the mother said.

"Kids? Kids *know* this is a ripoff," Coakley said. "Kids tell me— almost every time, this is what they tell you first—that the first question they get asked at these hospitals is, 'Who's your dad insured with?' Not 'Hi,' not 'How'ya doing?', not even 'What's your name?' That's one of the reasons the recovery rates at these expensive places are so minimal. These kids are coming from some sort of setting that's usually hypocritical anyway, a broken home or whatever, and then they get put into this environment that they know full well is a ripoff, where people are not leveling with them. They know why they're there—because of the insurance money. And they see this is just one more step in a series of things that just aren't right about life."

As Coakley's activities got local attention, a newspaper followed up with some tough reporting. In 1987, the *Palm Beach Post* found that some private psychiatric hospitals appeared to be abusing the Baker Act—the Florida law providing for involuntary hospitalization of mentally ill people who exhibit "clear and convincing" evidence of imminent danger—to facilitate the commitment of adolescents. The county mental-health office also reported numerous complaints from relatives of patients whom Fair Oaks had refused to discharge.

But the radio interviews stopped after Silverman, who had relished the fury that Coakley's by now weekly stints produced, left for a job with a radio station in Arizona.

With a lack of interest on the part of state and county regulators, the story largely died in south Florida, not to be revived elsewhere until more aggressive state officials got angry in Texas four years later.

Meanwhile, the Lions Club never saw Coakley's slide presentation. In a memo distributed to employees on July 23, 1987, the hospital's administrator, Mark Schneider, instructed staff members to keep Coakley off hospital grounds, denouncing "his rhetoric" about psychiatric profiteering as an attempt "to stir up public reaction."

In Texas, another whistle-blower with no ax to grind, Russell D. Durrett, knew how Coakley felt.

With nearly a quarter century running the accounting office of hospitals and other health-care companies. Durrett thought he had seen it all. But his eight months as the chief comptroller at Twin Lakes Hospital, an NME psychiatric hospital in Denton, Texas, near Fort Worth, were a genuine revelation to an accountant who believed his job description included warning his employer when the numbers didn't quite add up and refusing to certify fraud.

"Violations of Medicare regulations, state regulations, Internal Revenue Service regulations, violations of accepted business practices—this was definitely a part of health care that I hadn't seen before," said Durrett, a reserved man in his early fifties who knew that going public with his complaints about his employer would not only get him fired, but might also permanently brand him as a troublemaker in a close-knit business. Nevertheless, he felt that his professional ethics, not to mention his personal sense of social responsibility, outweighed the risks. So he decided to tell about it.

"The bottom line was the driving force behind almost every decision," Durrett said.

Having worked mostly in acute-care general hospitals, Durrett was surprised when he started work at Twin Lakes by the huge profit potential in psychiatric hospitals. Like others who eventually blew the whistle on psychiatric-hospital fraud, he first was fascinated, then quickly grew suspicious, while musing about the remarkable cash flow.

"The cost to get into the psychiatric-hospital business is cheap," he said. He figured that at the end of the eighties, a hundred-bed psychiatric hospital could still be built for less than $7 million. (To build a general hospital of comparable size would cost more than $45 million.) Psychiatric hospitals also require less professional staff and have far fewer regulations and medical guidelines to restrict their operations or add costs. Furthermore, "bad debts and charity care are almost nonexistent" at private psychiatric hospitals. "A psychiatric hospital can collect approximately 92 percent of its charges; a medical/surgical hospital is lucky to collect 55 percent.

"The money was just phenomenal," Durrett said, which would have been fine if the company had been selling appliances or fried chicken, but was not so fine for a firm whose business was providing psychiatric care in a hospital.

He was impressed by how the argot of marketing pervaded the institution; every employee was expected to be a recruiter of patients. For executives, the work week was filled with "admission and intervention" sessions, gatherings where top managers poured over constantly updated reports on patient censuses, the status of leads obtained from telephone responses to ads, and the performance of the extensive network of community based "referral" contacts—the counselors, clerics, and cops, among others, from whom new patients were obtained. The admissions office had put open telephone hot lines—no dialing required—directly into the booking areas of local police stations.

At formal weekly marketing meetings, "each person was asked to review their contacts for the previous week and any admissions from their contacts," Durrett recalled. "Everyone had a number of 'cold' contacts that they were required to make each week. There were subgroups within the marketing committee that were assigned to such areas as high schools and intermediate schools. Elementary schools were a separate group. Employee-assistance programs were another.

"The hospital paid for counselors at various schools—these counselors were school-district employees, not employees of the hospital." Schoolkids were especially valued patients, since they were usually hospitalized because their parents wanted them to be. "It was easy to extend the discharge date by not allowing the patient to show progress in their treatment program," he said.

Staff psychiatrists were expected to be key team players. "Any time that a psychiatrist was recruited," Durrett said, "the psychiatrist was given a title as a unit medical director." At Twin Lakes, psychiatrist salaries—for a ten-hour-a-week job—ranged from $10,000 to $15,000 a month. (Durrett signed the paychecks.) Since they maintained private practices as well, many psychiatrists also received reimbursement for their off-site office rent and staff. Private practices were a major referral channel for the hospital. A psychiatrist admitting one of his or her own patients into the hospital had an added incentive, Durrett said: "The physician could then bill a daily charge—usually a hundred to a hundred and fifty dollars for seeing the patient, as well as separate charges for any therapy. There were many occasions when a single physician would have over twenty-five patients in the hospital."

Psychiatry as a profession has traditionally been near the bottom of the medical specialties in average salary. For a psychiatrist willing to be "with the program," working at a private psychiatric hospital could be the road to riches. At Twin Lakes and many other private hospitals, psychiatrists were routinely making between $600,000 and $900,000 a year, Durrett said.

As the controller, he questioned odd "consulting" contracts on the payroll. He was told that one consultant, a nationally known authority on addiction, received $4,000 a month just for dropping the "Twin Lakes" name in his speeches to civic and social groups around the country.

"All the measurements for success of the hospital were financial," Durrett said. "The bottom line was the driving force behind almost every decision."

Of course, a controller's job by definition concerns the bottom line, including "telling the people you work for the things they need to be watching out for." This was where Durrett hit his major roadblocks.

When he arrived, the hospital was expanding rapidly—it had just grown in one year from sixty-eight to 104 beds. The new beds increased the pressure to keep customers coming through the door and to make sure they could all pay their bills. All hospital front offices are engrossed in insurance matters, but Durrett had never seen anything like the dedication that Twin Lakes applied to the task. Senior managers met weekly to review "insurance remaining reports" prepared by the accounting department, which detailed every patient's insurance coverage and the amount remaining. This, then, would determine who was "cured," Durrett said.

"Discharge planning would normally only be discussed for those patients who were running out of insurance coverage," Durrett said. Patients with limited benefits—say, twenty-eight days of hospitalization a year for alcohol or drug treatment—were scheduled for discharge on the day the benefits ran out.

"The hospital paid for counselors at various schools," he said. "There was a team assigned within the marketing group that targeted the various schools in our market area."

Insurance benefits offered by major local employers, such as Texas Instruments, were carefully scrutinized. For example, Texas Instruments offered generous psychiatric benefits of up to $50,000 a year. And a new year meant new opportunity: "Once a new benefit year started, patients were contacted to see if they required additional services," said Durrett.

He soon decided that there was a phrase to describe what he was observing: "criminally fraudulent." Routinely, Durrett said, patients were billed for sessions they never attended. "It was not uncommon for the adolescent program to have eight therapy sessions a day and also to have the patient attend high school classes, in-house, for a half a day."

In fact, sometimes the money came in such quantities that it was an embarrassment. "While I was at Twin Lakes it became clear that the [NME] hospitals within this region were making too much profit." At month's end, Durrett said, the "profit" for each hospital would be set at NME's psychiatric-division corporate headquarters, and "the regional vice president of finance would call each hospital and inform the hospital where to create additional expenses if the profit was too high."

For example, "Twin Lakes was budgeted to make $2.7 million profit for the fiscal year June 1987 to May 1988. The actual profit was $4.2 million," even with $670,000 in what Durrett called "ghost expenses" added in. Overall, said the former controller, "the amount of expenses that cannot be supported by proper expense documents had to be in excess of several million dollars for NME hospitals in our region alone."

One reason for this strategy, said Durrett, was to indicate a well-managed, steady rise in profitability, thus disguising from Wall Street analysts the suddenly volatile conditions that buffeted the industry at the end of the eighties.

He was astonished that the invoices and tax statements sailed through without a hitch. "We would crank out a $75,000 bill and never see an insurance auditor," he said with a chuckle. "And the IRS? Never a question about those expenses."

Though it was not interested in "charity" patients, the hospital did show its concern for some unemployed patients who suddenly lost their insurance benefits: According to Durrett, Twin Lakes paid the premium itself so that the coverage could continue.

"We'd get a postal money order so it would not show our name as making the payments for the patient," he explained. The payment would be sent anonymously, the insurance would be verified as still being in effect, and the hospital would "then turn around and bill [the insurance companies] anywhere from twenty-five thousand to fifty thousand dollars, Durrett said. "I believe this was a system-wide practice [in NME's psychiatric division] and not just our region."

Durrett, who left his job at Twin Lakes in the summer of 1989, was certain that the abuses he saw were not confined to Texas, or even to NME. In a 1992 letter to Representative Patricia Schroeder, chairwoman of the House Select Committee on Children, Youth and Families, Durrett said: "At the monthly regional meetings, the discussion always included what had worked at other hospitals in other regions. . . . The practices that were used in our hospitals were not isolated to our hospitals but . . . could be found in every hospital in our region . . . and most likely could be found in the other for-profit psychiatric chains. . . . Even the freestanding not-for-profit facilities were using many of the same practices."

CHAPTER THIRTEEN

....

As he would be the first to admit Duard Bok was no diplomat, even in the best of times. And for a staff psychiatrist in a corporate psychiatric-hospital chain in 1991, the best of times were fading fast.

In the early months of 1991, after he decided that his employers expected staff doctors to keep the beds full or else, the fifty-one-year-old Bok decided to confront the issue in his own characteristic way.

"Sleazebags!" he bellowed about his superiors, as nurses scurried for cover and other less emboldened psychiatrists hurried off to drink their coffee elsewhere lest they be assumed to be part of an incipient mutiny. "A bunch of fucking sleazebags!" It did not mitigate the problem appreciably when Bok made it a point to concede, "Of course, this is a subjective assessment on my part."

Not that Bok had a problem with making money by selling his services. He wasn't a medical missionary, after all; he was a modern psychiatrist, a very successful one, a man known as one of the top alcoholism and drug-addiction specialists in the Dallas–Fort Worth megalopolis in the 1980s, the kind of physician-businessman who could speak proudly of providing "appropriate diagnosis and service for a respectable, reasonable profit."

207

But he decided things had gone too far when *On War*, the seminal nineteenth-century military treatise by Prussian general Karl von Clausewitz, was held up as a model for discussion at medical staff meetings. Clausewitz's theory of an all-out assault on the enemy's territory, troops, resources, and will to fight was fine for war, but Bok considered it inappropriate as a model for attitudes toward potential hospital patients. Likewise, another in-house favorite, *Guerrilla Marketing*, a popular eighties how-to manual by a former advertising executive, Jay Conrad Levinson, was perhaps reasonable in advising total ruthlessness, cunning, stealth, and resourcefulness to sell potato chips or hamburgers—but questionable, Bok decided, as an approach to psychiatry.

"It seemed to me they took those warlike strategies and became totally ruthless, and the only thing was the profit," Bok recalled. "People shifted from the status of patients, in my opinion, to the status of commodity. Patients to some degree have always been commodities—but they now shifted totally to commodities. They became dehumanized."

Sunbelt sprawls like the Dallas–Fort Worth region, basking in the goodwill of the Reagan era, were good places in the 1980s to practice psychiatry, a profession that tends to prosper in tune with the economy. The hospitals were full of patients, many of them referred there by a cozy but competent network of medical specialists of all stripes in the area.

So business was good—but it was never good enough for the voracious demands of the quarterly earnings report. And once the lengths of stay began to drop with the corporate cutbacks at the tail end of the eighties, life in the psychiatric hospital was one constant marketing rally. Bok's employer, NME, ran a tight ship, and the storm clouds were dark on the horizon.

Bok readily concedes that he went along without protest for a while. But the old-style independent-minded psychiatrists were a dying breed, he decided, and their successors were frightening—

compliant young doctors hungry for riches; corporate soldiers ready to march on command. Bok admits frankly that among his motivations for rebellion was the fact that his own income began to decline.

By the early spring of 1991, Bok was manifesting a tone of outright contempt toward two NME hospitals in the Dallas–Fort Worth area, Psychiatric Institute of Fort Worth and Bedford Meadows Hospital, where he was employed as a medical program director. Since Bok—a blustery South African who took no guff from anyone, who cursed like a sailor when confronted by what he regarded as stupidity, and who was regarded even in the most placid of times as a loose cannon on the deck of the bureaucracy—was already the most feared psychiatrist on either hospital's staff, this made many people very uneasy.

Bok had a thriving private practice and had been affiliated with hospitals owned by NME since the middle of the 1980s. It wasn't a perfect situation, but Bok regarded the marketing as falling within his own "threshold of tolerance." At first, atmosphere wasn't rapacious, he said: "It wasn't crazy, it wasn't out of control. There was a little corner-cutting and sometimes they did keep people in the hospital maybe a little longer than they should have in terms of medical justification, and maybe they did admit a few people where they could have used a less restrictive form of treatment."

Trouble developed after a new administrator came in, a marketing whiz, Bok said, under orders to "bring up the census." He did just that, through unremitting marketing efforts. For a while, with new medical fees rolling in with the new patients, all was well, though Bok and other physicians already affiliated with the hospital believed that the local psychiatric market was pretty well saturated.

The hospital launched a successful campaign to hire as "consultants" a large number of outside psychiatrists in the region, Bok said. "They told them specifically, not obliquely: 'Now you are on our payroll. We want you to refer to us.' They captured the referral sources of the psychiatrists." This, he felt, had the effect of making the entire regional psychiatric establishment play ball.

Bok sent a patient from his private practice to one of the hospitals. Just before Christmas, Bok said, he ordered the man discharged, planning to continue treating him as an outpatient. "They went to this guy behind my back and said, 'Well, we think you need more inpatient treatment,' " he said. "The guy owed about four thousand dollars on his deductible, which the insurance wouldn't pick up. They said, 'Okay, if you stay in for three or four more weeks, we'll waive the deductible and any further deductible—and you'll get better treatment."

Outraged at what he regarded as interference in his medical prerogatives, Bok let it be known at staff meetings what he thought about the way the business was being run. "I raised my voice, pounded on the table, and said what they were doing wasn't appropriate." The response, he said, was "snickering. I would get upset and talk about it, they would snicker."

Bok did have his supporters, especially among the "grunts"— duty shrinks and nurses—who cheered him on, though they did so anonymously.

Bok escalated his attacks, openly marveling at the spectacular new breakthroughs in biopsychiatry that enabled all of these patients to be cured on the very day their insurance ran out. Actually, he marveled at the ability of some patients to get well despite their treatment. He conveyed to staff psychiatrists, psychologists, and licensed counselors his contempt for their complicity in bounty-hunting programs. Corporate profit needs were usurping the role of the physician in determining treatment for patients—and this with the assistance of professionals who were terrified of the corporation, he said. On rounds some days, Bok would come across a patient whose discharge he had ordered—and be confronted by a staff therapist begging him to keep the patient hospitalized until the insurance benefits ran out. Again and again, Bok said, he came across drug-addicted or alcoholic patients who had been "deceived" into inpatient treatment by counselors associated with twelve-step programs like Alcoholics Anonymous, but secretly affiliated with various psychiatric hospitals.

At medical staff meetings, Bok railed that his and other physicians' signatures had sometimes been "forged" on medical records so as to keep patients in. He ridiculed several other physicians for admitting patients with "multiple-personality disorders" without the expertise to treat them and for rolling over patients from one diagnosis to another, to exhaust benefits under each. He was especially incensed by the use of rage reduction therapy, in which children were held down and then taunted until they exploded in fury. Bok demanded that the psychiatrist in charge of the program be fired.

"If a police officer saw an adult doing that in the front yard they'd pick them up for child abuse," he complained. "Here, we're charging for it and calling it therapy." The hospital changed the name of the treatment to "trust development therapy." Bok raised other objections to children's programs; for example, he asserted that there was a practice of amply dosing children with psychoactive drugs, then intentionally depriving them of sleep so they would react in a way that fit diagnoses of depression and irritability. Bok went home one night and pounded out a forty-page memo detailing his complaints, and spent hours faxing it to local newspapers, the regional office of the state child protective services agency, and the Tarrant County district attorney.

In April 1991, his relationships with colleagues badly strained—calling them pimps and sellouts did not help—Bok had his lawyer deliver to the hospital administrator a formal letter expressing his "deep concerns" about some of the hospital's practices.

Perhaps worst of all, Bok said, he began discussing with several hospital program counselors the idea of setting up a private group to provide alternative, inexpensive addiction treatment in the kind of medically supervised outpatient program that Bok firmly believed was the most effective way to treat the vast majority of alcoholism and substance-abuse cases. Now, he heard, he had gone too far, especially since he had stopped admitting patients.

"My attitude by then was, 'Fuck 'em. Come after me and make my day,' " Bok said.

They did. At a special executive committee meeting at Psychiatric Institute of Fort Worth, Bok was declared to be mentally ill. On July 30, the hospital sent a letter to the Texas Medical Association's impaired physicians committee, which evaluates complaints against physicians and has the power to revoke a medical license, describing Bok as "likely impaired." The letter accused Bok of dereliction in administrative duties, interfering in other physicians' affairs, and displaying "arrogance," with an attitude toward fellow staff psychiatrists that "could be described as belittling and condescending."

Furthermore, said the hospital's letter, Bok's "deteriorating conduct and behavior," was illustrated by his failing to renew the annual federal DEA permit that physicians need to prescribe certain classes of controlled drugs, including many psychiatric medications. "Unless he has subsequently and therefore unknown to us either had a spontaneous remission of his condition or has allowed someone to assist him professionally," the letter to the medical board continued, Bok was not considered to be a "capable" physician.

The letter added that the hospital administration was prepared to assist in any inquiry into Bok's alleged impairment, and any future efforts "to rehabilitate this man" to an "appropriate level" of competence.

Bok said he found several true statements in the letter. He had indeed temporarily forgotten to renew the DEA permit that allowed him to write prescriptions for certain addictive drugs, because he seldom prescribed such drugs. The permit was routinely renewed, but he did not think the oversight was a symptom of mental illness, not even according to the *DSM*.

And he *had* been contemptuous. Laughing, he read from the letter: " '*The form of these manifested behaviors was an arrogant manner toward the professional staff. . . .*' " "That, actually, is quite true. I really did believe that they were assholes. I guess you can fault me for having that position, because it showed. '*His attitude toward fellow physicians could be described as belittling and condescending. . . .*' True again. So what? As they got worse, I got more and more critical. I'm proud of the attitude I communicated to them. That makes me crazy?"

But the letter made Bok think of a marketing director he had known at one hospital who had defected to a competitor. Baseless rumors that the man had been a drug abuser arose, seemingly spontaneously. He remembered another former colleague, a caring nurse who was labeled as being clinically "co-dependent" after she defied a superior and persisted in spending extra time comforting a terrified five-year-old patient.

Word got around, of course, that Bok had been reported to the state medical board as impaired. Like police stations, hospitals are notorious rumor mills, with embellishments left behind like stale coffee from work shift to work shift. One that astounded Bok had him supposedly roaring into the medical-records room and furiously tearing apart patient files. Another, especially ridiculous from his vantage point, was that he had been committed to another psychiatric hospital for six weeks and "cured."

Bok began to question the ethical underpinnings and philosophical soundness of psychiatry, especially as practiced in a for-profit hospital. "It seems to me now, from being around large psychiatric organizations and psychiatrists in general, if you take a stand which is in opposition to where they are, and they have no other recourse, the recourse they resort to is to say you're crazy. Not only in this country but in every other country, if all else fails, psychiatrists are programmed to call people who disagree with their position mentally ill."

Two things were fairly clear to Bok: He was boxed in, and he was on his own. "If you get angry, they say that's symptomatic and evidence of psychiatric deficiency. If you're quiet about it, you're indifferent. If you react, there's evidence of instabiity." But the hospital misjudged his tenacity, he said. "The issues coming to light throughout the psychiatric-hospital business were not just casual occurrences. These were massive, serious perpetrations against patients. And it was systemic.

"They expect you to keep quiet. They count on you to worry about your reputation, protect your position. And my response to that was, 'Forget it.' " He decided to go as public as he could. "I called everybody in the media to bolster my position when I had no constituency." A few newspaper stories were written.

In August, the hospital fired Bok. At an impairment hearing in October, Psychiatric Institute of Fort Worth's medical director, Dr. Virgil Cox, testified that he believed Bok suffered from a "bi-polar personality disorder which impairs his judgment and adversely affects his ability to practice medicine." Furthermore, said Cox, "he has displayed the attitude that only he knows what's wrong with the hospital or the hospital programs." However, under questioning, Cox conceded that he could identify only three specific examples of Bok's "disordered" behavior over six years and had not mentioned them to colleagues at the time.

Bok had claimed that administrators pressured psychiatrists to revise diagnoses so patients could be kept in the hospital until insurance limits were exhausted.

Bok ultimately got a call from Senator Frank Tejeda's office. They had to phone long distance, however, because Bok and his wife, Margaret, who is also a well-known psychiatrist, had moved to Alabama with their son, who had been taunted at school that his father was a lunatic.

The psychiatrist Peter Breggin, a leading critic of his profession, also was hauled before a state medical board—Maryland's, in 1987—and had to defend his license after he criticized drug therapy during an appearance on Oprah Winfrey's television show. The complaint against Breggin had been brought by NAMI, the National Alliance for the Mentally Ill, which is closely tied to corporate psychiatry. Breggin kept his medical license—the complaint was dismissed as an attempt to abrogate his First Amendment rights to speak freely—but the case was widely publicized within the psychiatric profession, and the message was clear. Still, though psychiatrists have long known that rebellion has its price, some continue to pay it.

Like Duard Bok, Dr. Robert F. Stuckey was a prominent figure in addiction treatment. But by the middle of 1985, Stuckey, who had been medical director of the important alcoholism unit at NME's Fair Oaks Hospital in Summit, New Jersey, for nearly ten years, had finally had enough. He decided that profits were all the hospital cared about.

Stuckey, too, berated his colleagues, storming out of a hospital board meeting after telling his fellow members: "You are only interested in money. I have never once heard any discussion by this board about patient care and ways to improve it. Here, I only am pushed to compel the system to procure more money. It is unconsionable, and I resign." Fellow board members were all the more aghast because Stuckey himself was one of the leading medical developers of for-profit addiction-treatment facilities in the United States.

Six years later, Stuckey was still furious, especially since New Jersey state regulators, insurance-company officials, and the New Jersey news media had seemed uninterested in his repeated attempts to voice complaints until Texas officials began exposing the psychiatric-hospital scandal in 1991. Stuckey said he had been ready for years with a ferocious indictment of the abuses he said he had witnessed at Fair Oaks.

"I was constantly pressured to keep patients longer and order more lab testing," he recalled. The hospital insisted, he said, on conducting lab tests that he considered to be unnecessary and ridiculous, including sperm counts for every male patient, and "street drug" testing even for the elderly.

In ten years, Stuckey watched the daily room rate at Fair Oaks rise from $150 to over $1,000 a day, with corresponding hikes in medical-service fees and other costs. In his last year on the staff, he became uneasy about what he later described as the hospital's "frightening ability" to prosper from "demoralized, vulnerable, confused, and very often gullible" patients who were seeking help for emotional problems or addictions.

Interest in insurance benefits was both intense and ceaseless. "They were absolute geniuses at diagnosing insurance," Stuckey said with amazement. When a prospective patient contacted Fair Oaks, his or her insurance coverage was thoroughly researched. Once the patient was admitted, insurance was regularly reviewed to ascertain "how the hospital could legally acquire every dollar possible that was still available that day, on that policy," Stuckey remembered. "The patient usually received the diagnosis that matched the category with the most money available to it."

Stuckey recalled initially becoming suspicious when he began noticing familiar faces back in the hospital, in another ward, after he had ordered them discharged from the alcoholism unit. He discovered that the hospital was designing new diagnoses for patients who had exhausted their coverage for alcoholism but still had coverage left for, say, depression. "I'd watch them being moved from unit to unit, and after a while it became clear to me that insurance was what was behind it. Once the benefits were used up in one area, they'd get another diagnosis and shift them to a new program that still had benefits." Sadly, he concluded that "the primary function of the hospital, a function so important that it rendered all other functions incidental, was to extract every single penny possible from the patients."

CHAPTER FOURTEEN

....

IT HAD ALL GROWN DANGEROUSLY QUICKLY. INEVITABLY, THERE would be a shakeout in the psychiatric industry, just as there had been in the corporate general-hospital business in the mid-eighties. Even though construction costs for a psychiatric hospital were far less than those for a general hospital, all of those new beds were not as easy to keep occupied by paying customers in what had begun to look like a grossly overbuilt market.

"Some of the smaller companies are running out of capital," Loren B. Shook, the executive vice president of CPC, told *Modern Healthcare* in 1987. It had been a big year for CPC, which then had thirty-two hospitals, plus fourteen new ones under construction.

At NME, Norman A. Zober, the hard-driving head of the psychiatric-hospitals division, then had ten hospitals under construction, which would soon bring the total number to fifty-seven, and counting. He remained sanguine. "There are still a lot of underserved areas in the United States. The need is staggering," he opined.

But so were the costs, and those who paid them were beginning to squeal.

For employers, psychiatric and substance-abuse benefits had

become major expenses. Furthermore, there didn't seem to be any reasonable ceiling on psychiatric costs, which were rising way out of proportion to employee medical costs in general—and by 1984 such costs were claiming 24 percent of corporate America's pretax profits. In 1992, health-care costs averaged $3,968 per employee.

That was before psychiatric costs began climbing at even higher rates. A national benefits-consulting firm, A. Foster Higgins, found in its annual survey of corporate benefit plans that for companies employing more than five thousand people, the cost of psychiatric and substance-abuse treatment rose 47 percent from 1988 to 1989. Overall, mental-health costs for all U.S. employers shot up 27 percent between 1987 and 1989, according to the Employee Benefits Research Institute. While only a small percentage of employees and dependents were then making mental-health claims, such benefits are among the most expensive medical outlays provided— even though there was no consensus on their effectiveness. Still, a survey cited by *The Wall Street Journal* put the average *per case* billing for psychiatric care for an adolescent at $18,000—far more than most serious medical treatments such as major surgery.

By 1990, mental-health and substance-abuse treatment costs accounted for "as much as 20 to 30 percent of an employer's total medical costs" at some firms, according to a report by the Health Insurance Association of America. The prices of psychiatric drugs, the mainstays of modern treatment, were also skyrocketing. According to the organization Common Cause, the price of the popular sedative Halcion, made by Upjohn, rose 75 percent between 1986 and 1991.

Something had to give. Alarmed by runaway inflation in employee health benefits, businesspeople who typically spoke of the free-enterprise system with the reverence of nuns describing the Vatican found themselves in the unfamiliar position of advocating increased government control of health care.

When the economic boom of the eighties flattened at the end of the decade, major employers finally acknowledged a problem that smaller employers had been grumbling about for years: An extraordinary number of mental-health benefits were being provided (often as a requirement by state law). Of the various service-specific health benefits (such as eye care, Pap smears, dental care, and the like), inpatient psychiatric care had become the most common employee health-insurance benefit, with alcoholism and drug-abuse care close behind. Corporate benefits managers began to consider that about 85 percent of the money spent on mental-health benefits was going to inpatient hospitalization, despite the fact that only a small percentage of people—the accepted figure even in the late eighties was less than 15 percent—who seek treatment for mental illness or substance abuse need to be in a hospital. Benefits managers had on their desks review after review indicating that inpatient treatment for alcoholism or drug abuse was no better than (far less expensive) outpatient treatment.

By the late eighties, many small and medium-sized employers had already adopted some kind of new controls on psychiatric and substance-abuse hospitalization. Chiefly these were limits on the annual number of days of hospitalization. Some firms, such as Ameritrust, reported immediate and remarkable improvement. Adopting a form of "managed care," with close controls on admissions, Ameritrust cut its annual addiction-treatment costs by a third in 1988, even while providing treatment to 11 percent more people.

Big companies were slower to act because it was harder for them to evaluate individual cases. But as costs got out of control at the end of the decade, major employers put on the brakes, and the psychiatric industry suddenly had to scramble and market even harder just to keep the beds full. This, in hindsight, has been identified as the catalyst that changed what had been "merely" unethical conduct in the psychiatric industry into, in some cases, criminal conduct.

In some companies, painful reassessments were made of those $30,000-a-month sojourns for alcoholism or drug-addiction treatment. "Companies with liberal and enlightened policies like us found we were sending some of our people to rehab two and three times," said a corporate benefits manager of a large Philadelphia company. "Finally, it came down to, 'Hey, what kind of a bang are we getting for these bucks?' Frankly, I think some managers were using employee-assistance committees to ship problems out the door for a while rather than deal with them as personnel matters. In some departments, it was looked on almost like detention in high school."

In 1990, two major U.S. employers, AT&T and IBM, set the pace for reducing psychiatric costs by organizing in-house health-care systems. IBM, alarmed by 20-percent-a-year increases in these costs, hired an outside management firm to operate networks of psychiatrists, psychologists, and other therapists at treatment centers to provide mental-health and substance-abuse care for 700,000 IBM employees and dependents in the United States.

Not long afterward, General Motors, which had been paying as much as $80 million a year just for addiction treatment, hired an outside company to manage its mental-health benefits covering about 1.5 million employees and retirees. Xerox also tightened the limits on psychiatric and substance-abuse hospitalization for its 55,000 workers.

The federal government, the nation's largest employer, finally lumbered into response, instituting tighter controls on psychiatric reimbursement. In 1989, the federal government had spent more than $360 million to provide inpatient mental-health and substance-abuse treatment for its three million civilian employees. This figure doesn't include CHAMPUS outlays—$613 million in 1989 for mental-health benefits for military dependents and retirees (an increase of 126 percent in just five years). CHAMPUS, which spent nearly $500 million of that $613 million to reimburse psychiatric hospitals for inpatient care, also put limits on yearly increases in charges and set a daily maximum rate for hospitalization.

Overbuilt, deeply in debt, beset by competitors, burdened with investors who had come to anticipate 30 percent annual returns, psychiatric-hospital corporations were suddenly confronted with basic economic realities. Occupancy rates at many of their hospitals began to drop.

NME's 1991 annual report sounded a note of concern about the decline in the average number of days patients stayed in the hospital: "The rise of managed care and utilization review caused significant declines in average length of stay"—to twenty-four days in 1991, down sharply from thirty-one days in 1988. At Charter Medical's eighty-two psychiatric hospitals, the average length of stay fell to 20.4 days in 1991 (it had been twenty-seven days three years earlier). As lengths of stay declined, overall annual occupancy rates also sagged. At the four major psychiatric chains, occupancy rates in 1991 were down: to less than 50 percent at CPC; just over 50 percent at Charter and HCA; just over 70 percent at NME.

Naturally, ambitious expansion plans in the industry were scuttled or put on indefinite hold.

In 1991, according to the annual survey by *Modern Healthcare* magazine, the number of beds operated by private, investor-owned psychiatric hospitals grew only 0.8 percent, to a total of 35,389. Charter actually reported a net drop in the number of beds—from 7,951 in 1990 to 7,449 in 1991.

The psychiatric profession, inexorably tied by now to the hospital business, was worried. To handle calls from psychiatrists alarmed about having their decisions second-guessed by corporate oversight managers, the APA installed its own crisis hot line—an 800 number for members to call for advice.

But for the hospitals, driven by marketing, the solution was obvious: If the customers were staying for less time, find more customers. The critical necessity of doing that was often made clear in no uncertain terms.

In September of 1990, Michael J. Safran, a vice president and regional administrator in NME's psychiatric hospitals division, distributed a memo to the division's senior vice presidents in advance of a regional planning meeting. The memo presented statistics indicating a failure to meet preset goals for patient censuses and average lengths of stay. Among the problem "issues" underscored were concerns about falling admission rates, lack of "discharge planning control," "poor length-of-stay management," "precipitous" discharges of patients by attending psychiatrists, and "weak defense" of hospitalization under pressure from third-party payers.

Hospital program directors, who are the psychiatrists who run major treatment programs, and "intake" staff, the admissions and marketing people, were exhorted to be always mindful of daily admissions "goals." Administrators were advised to replace program directors who were unwilling to comply.

Denial, long a buzzword in psychiatry, had taken on an entirely new meaning in the executive suite. A major worry was the increasing number of denials of full-treatment authorization by newly vigilant third-party insurance payers. In response, NME was setting up a "Denial Hot Line" to provide tips on how to avoid denials. The memo stressed the importance of physician diagnoses, in a way that strongly suggested NME psychiatrists had better understand clearly who they worked for:

> The significance of denials is constantly reinforced to administrators, controllers, business office staff, intake staff, program directors and through them to the Medical Directors and attending [physicians]. The intent is to prevent or minimize the possibility of denials, and therefore the following approach will be taken: [in the event an insurance company denies approval] . . . go up the approval chain, using the Medical Director, if necessary.

And then there was the matter of Texas, where some investigators were so angry they were now talking about throwing people in jail.

CHAPTER FIFTEEN

....

ACTUALLY, INVESTIGATORS IN NEW JERSEY HAD BEEN INTER-ested in psychiatric hospitals well before the Harrell boy's ordeal outraged legislators in Texas. Looking into allegations that had swirled around NME's Fair Oaks Hospital in Summit since Dr. Stuckey had begun making noises years before, New Jersey Insurance Department investigators finally decided to begin "kicking ass and taking names," as one investigator, Dick Mason, a former organized-crime task force detective, would put it. The department's fraud division confronted NME with detailed evidence of questionable insurance claims from Fair Oaks Hospital, and demanded that the hospital pay a penalty of $2 million.

The insurance department backed off, however, in the face of NME lawyers, who insisted on detailed proof of intent on every aspect of each disputed claim. Finally in the spring of 1991, New Jersey agreed to a settlement of $400,000 from NME on the Fair Oaks charges. This was the largest consent settlement ever assessed by the department. But NME successfully insisted that the agreement not include any admission of guilt, and that it therefore be kept secret under the terms of a New Jersey statute that blocks authorities from formally notifying licensing authorities—in this case the state health department—in the event of a consent agreement in which wrongdoing is not admitted.

The agreement, signed in May 1991, denied fraud and admitted only that "certain human or computer errors may have resulted in the mistaken submission of claims for non-reimbursable items." The hospital said it was paying $350,000—the other $50,000 was paid by an affiliate—"to avoid needless legal expenses and to reimburse the state for its cost of investigation." The state insurance department did not put out a press release announcing the settlement, as would be routine in such a record settlement. The New Jersey Insurance Department received the payment of $400,000 on May 17.

The secret deal with New Jersey soon unraveled. While Senator Tejeda's office was just gearing up in Texas, the *Palm Beach Post*, the newspaper that had done the best job following up on the charges about psychiatric hospitals made years earlier by Bill Coakley, broke the story of the Fair Oaks settlement with New Jersey— prompting red-faced officials in New Jersey to quickly announce that they had decided to continue their investigation, and prompting NME to demand its money back, since the deal had been breached.

Meanwhile, the 1991 NME annual report, ready at the end of the summer, enthused about "record earnings," and hailed the psychiatric division's "23 percent increase in total admissions" and its occupancy rate, "higher than any other major psychiatric hospital company." It added: "Demand for psychiatric hospital services remains high" because of "the steady rise in demand for quality psychiatric services." However, the report did cite increased pressure from insurance companies.

In late September, Eamer, the chairman, told shareholders at the annual meeting: "We believe that NME is stronger financially today than at any time in its history," and predicted continued robust growth. He did not seem outwardly concerned about the rumblings in Texas. Still, Texas was a problem not only for NME, but for the psychiatric industry in general—and it wasn't going away as easily as New Jersey had.

For investigators in Texas, prompted into action by Senator Tejeda's office, had been hard at work all through the spring and summer of 1991, and they were kicking up a storm that would soon batter the psychiatric-hospital business as nothing else in its brief and profitable history had done.

A week after Jeramy Harrell was let out of the hospital, Tejeda had enlisted the state mental-health and mental-retardation division to pull the records of emergency-detention admissions at Colonial Hills. On May 17, the agency had issued a report that Sector One security officers in Bexar County had indeed been doing emergency detentions "based on hearsay or double-hearsay information. . . . We are concerned that under this arrangement, individuals may be denied liberty for monetary gain on the part of Sector One and the contract agents." The report recommended the district attorney conduct his investigation into both Sector One and Dr. Bowlan, the psychiatrist who had signed Jeramy Harrell's admission orders.

Meanwhile, Dr. Bowlan had resigned from the staff of Colonial Hills. On May 2, the state Board of Medical Examiners had canceled his temporary license to practice medicine in Texas, charging him with having forged certain documents he filed in connection with his professional credentials to treat adolescents and children. Bowlan later moved to Oklahoma.

John Wayne Blanks was in trouble, too. On June 5, the Texas Board of Private Investigators filed four complaints against Sector One, its owner, and the employees, Saenz and Jones, who had taken the Harrell boy away. The complaints charged Blanks with fraud and deceit in filing the application for Jeramy's detention and charged Jones and Saenz with impersonating an officer. Blanks closed his company; his license was later revoked by the board. The Sector One guards who had apprehended the Harrell boy also were disciplined. Saenz had his license revoked; Jones was issued an official reprimand.

Meanwhile, the district attorney began looking into Colonial Hills Hospital as part of a criminal investigation.

Senator Tejeda was no longer using terms like "unethical practices." The phrase he chose now was "white-collar crime." He said, "Some of these psychiatric hospitals are getting more money with their briefcases, hiding behind their credentials, than a guy with a gun could get at a bank."

In the state capital, Senator Zaffirini, dismayed at "how widespread this is and how it reaches into our schools," followed up aggressively on Tejeda's initiative. In July, the state senate's Health and Human Service Subcomittee on Health Services, which she chaired, held a two-day "exploratory hearing" in San Antonio.

Tejeda led off, saying that what had happened to Jeramy Harrell was not an isolated case, that he and other legislators had been hearing endless horror stories, and that "the common denominator was that these individuals all were covered by insurance." These were frightened people, he said, who became "easy prey for those vultures" engaged in a "feeding frenzy for market share."

Then the Harrells took the stand.

Afterward, Senator Zaffirini and her two colleagues went to work in the legislature, pushing hard for emergency legislation to start tackling the problem. In September, thanks to the allegations spilling out of the San Antonio hearings, the state legislature passed a new law specifically outlawing bounty payments for referrals to hospitals. "They understand money. Let's talk money," Zaffirini had said, pushing to impose a stiff fine for every day a hospital was found to be in violation.

Meanwhile, the state attorney general, Dan Morales, who had taken office on January 1, had been puzzled about the huge amount of money that appeared to be going into hospital psychiatric treatment from the Texas Crime Victims Compensation Fund, which had paid out $22.2 million in benefits to five thousand Texas crime victims in 1990. Money for the fund comes from federal grants augmented by state assessments on criminal fines.

Payments to the four major chains had more than tripled, to $1.6 million, in two years, led by claims filed by NME's thirteen Texas hospitals.

On September 11, as investigators began gathering testimony throughout the state, Morales called a press conference to announce a lawsuit alleging that NME's psychiatric hospital subsidiary violated the state's newly enacted "medical kickback" law by paying referral fees for patients. "Frankly," Morales told reporters, "we fear we may just be scratching the surface, and that's the most troublesome notion of all." The attorney general said that NME paid $155,000 a month in operating expenses for a Fort Worth–area community referral service known as Recovery Line Inc., and also paid a "finder's fee" for referrals of "each victim of violent crime" who qualified for assistance under the state crime victims compensation fund. He said that some crime victims admitted to psychiatric hospitals were treated until they had exhausted the maximum $25,000 in individual benefits under the fund.

Responding to the suit, NME said, "We believe our facilities have made good-faith claims against the fund."

Morales had chosen a propitious time to act. That night, ABC's *Prime Time Live*, which had taken an interest in Zaffirini's July committee hearings, broadcast a report detailing the Harrell case and other questionable detentions of patients by Texas psychiatric hospitals. The American Psychiatric Association, which had kept quiet until the controversy spilled onto national television, reacted by issuing a statement that it was "gravely concerned" about "bullying outreach tactics" such as those being charged to psychiatric hospitals in Texas.

As soon as the charges were raised by the attorney general's office in September, Recovery Line fired three employees, citing rumors of solicitation of "bounty" payments from psychiatric hospitals. One favored tactic, another former employee revealed, was to attend Alcoholics Anonymous meetings, win the confidence of new members, ascertain their insurance benefits, and sell them into inpatient treatment programs such as those sponsored by psychiatric hospitals. One AA chapter in Fort Worth had even put a warning on its bulletin board: "Recovery Line—Stay Out!"

"They turned Alcoholics Anonymous into a whorehouse to support a billion-dollar industry," one woman told the *Houston Chronicle*, claiming that bounty hunters working for a private psychiatric hospital, upon discovering her liberal insurance coverage, duped her into entering the hospital when all she needed was "a few meetings" of AA.

Another case involved an unemployed single mother of three young teenagers who said she placed her children in a "Christian" children's shelter, but called Recovery Line when her thirteen-year-old daughter was molested there. Recovery Line advised hospitalization for all three children—ages twelve, thirteen, and fifteen—and said that the thirteen-year-old would qualify as a crime victim. Ultimately, the hospital, Psychiatric Institute of Fort Worth, claimed more than $30,000 for a total of fifty-four days of treatment.

Recovery Line had been operating in Texas out of seven offices, with forty-four employees. Max Tipton, who founded Recovery Line in 1990 as a toll-free referral-service hot line, admitted that NME had paid the agency's staff salaries and office expenses, but denied that any "quota" for referrals existed.

The attorney general, sympathizing with "law-abiding Texans traumatized at the hands of cold-blooded criminals one day and coldly calculating profiteers the next day," froze $10 million in unpaid claims on the Crime Victims Compensation Fund by psychiatric-hospital chains doing business in Texas. The claims frozen included $3.1 million by NME hospitals.

As former patients went public with their horror stories, others came forward with damaging information. Dr. Charles Overstreet, a psychiatrist on the staff of a nonprofit hospital in Fort Worth, told investigators that abuse in the region's psychiatric hospitals had been common knowledge among mental-health professionals. Some general hospitals simply showed the door to representatives of referral agencies like Recovery Line, who came around regularly like route salesman. Others did not. In one case, Dr. Overstreet recalled treating a man with a long history of alcoholism—a patient who was motivated to deal with his problem. The man's family called Overstreet to say that they had been approached by a "screening and referral service called Recovery Line," which "had made arrangements for him to be treated as an inpatient for chemical dependency, at no charge to the family." The physician questioned the wisdom of hospitalization; there were lots of effective outpatient chemical-dependency programs available, most relatively inexpensive, he told the family. "The thing that unnerved me a little bit was the vigor at which the Recovery Line people had sought this guy out and really lined all this up," Overstreet said. All of a sudden, a twenty-eight-day hospital stay was set up, fully covered by insurance. "All he had to do was show up."

However, when the patient arrived at Psychiatric Institute of Fort Worth to be admitted to the hospital's chemical-dependency program, he found himself instead hustled into the locked psychiatric ward, classified as a danger to himself. "He wanted to leave and they told him he couldn't, and that they were going to file to hold him" on a court order, said Overstreet, who marveled that a patient he had just seen, a man who had left his office requiring only reasonable treatment for alcoholism he was determined to conquer, had become a psychiatric emergency. "He got to that hospital and in a period of a few hours, he had all of a sudden been diagnosed as a danger to himself and had been locked up." It took a lawyer to get the man out.

A Recovery Line vice president, Wayne Mefford, a former sheriff's deputy, defended the service's record of providing referrals to people without insurance, telling the *Fort Worth Star Telegram*: "We don't advise people to go to PI. We might suggest it."

Mefford, a former county sheriff's officer, described Recovery

Line as a "community assessment and resource service," and denied that the company had to provide a certain number of patients a month to the hospital. "I am not a headhunter," said Mefford, who maintained that "eighty percent" of Recovery Line's business was devoted to providing emergency hospital transportation and other assistance to people without insurance. The funding from NME actually enabled the company to maintain 24-hour service to anyone who called, he said.

But others saw Recovery Line's practices differently. A lawsuit later filed against NME by eight major insurance companies, charging a "massive fraudulent scheme," said of Recovery Line: "Although nominally a separate entity, Recovery Line existed almost exclusively for the purpose of referring patients to NME psychiatric hospitals."

If the APA and the psychiatric industry thought things would quiet down in Texas, they were wrong. After the San Antonio "exploratory hearings," Senator Zaffirini wrote to the state lieutenant governor, Bob Bullock: "Our worst suspicions have been confirmed. . . . The problem is statewide and national." Bullock, who described himself as a recovering alcoholic, took an immediate interest in pursuing the case. He named Zaffirini, Moncrief, and Senator Chris Harris, a Democrat from Arlington, to an interim committee to conduct intensive hearings, traveling throughout Texas to elicit testimony from ordinary citizens about abuses in psychiatric hospitals. Moncrief was named to chair the hearings. The committee could draw on the talented investigative staff of the existing Health and Human Services Committee, and Moncrief gave the order: "Full steam ahead." Under direction of an energetic young administrator named Leslie Lemon, the committee staff coordinator, the four-member staff worked day and night for months lining up hundreds of witnesses and compiling background information for the senate.

Moncrief had been in fact a prominent supporter of legislation that provided for funding for alcohol- and drug-abuse treatment; indeed, he was a member of a community advisory board at CareUnit Hospital, a well-regarded private psychiatric hospital in Fort Worth. He quit the board upon being named to head the investigation.

Since a $7 billion industry was involved in these horror stories, the rumors finally began to unsettle Wall Street's health-care-stock analysts, who had so highly regarded psychiatric hospital stocks. Early in October, *The Wall Street Journal* reported that NME's psychiatric hospitals were under fraud investigation in five states. The Justice Department had begun a criminal investigation of CHAMPUS billings. (In 1990, the state with the most CHAMPUS claims was Texas, where CHAMPUS paid out $132 million for private mental-health services. California was next—the outlay there was $95 million—followed by Florida, Virginia, and Georgia. "Unfortunately, the mental-health industry is no different from any other business," U.S. Representative Beverly Byron had lamented during earlier hearings in Washington on overall CHAMPUS spending. "It will charge whatever the marketplace will bear.")

NME issued a press release in response to the clamor, announcing its own internal investigation. With that, investors bolted, afraid that the damage was already extensive. NME was the most actively traded stock on the New York Stock Exchange that day; the stock closed down more than $4, to $16.125 a share.

The forty-eight-year-old Zober, who had directed the growth of the psychiatric division from PIA headquarters in Washington, D.C., was the first to be thrown overboard. On October 8, NME announced that he had been placed on "indefinite leave of absence"—with pay—pending the results of the internal investigation. Some analysts speculated that Zober was being made a scapegoat; one, however, noted that his remaining on the payroll might at least ensure his discretion. In 1991, Zober received more than $2 million in salary, bonuses, and stock options; he continued to collect his pay through the 1992 fiscal year.

Eamer himself took his case to *The Wall Street Journal*, which on October 14 referred to NME as a company "long seen as the 'Mr. Clean' of its industry." Eamer told the newspaper that "we haven't done anything wrong" and threatened legal action against stock analysts who were busily scaling back once-rosy estimates of NME earnings. Eamer, who had shown up for the newspaper interview wearing a T-shirt that said, "I'm Not Arrogant—I'm Just Always Right," conceded that the psychiatric hospitals offered bonuses based on occupancy rates. And, he said, if NME's Texas hospitals did pay bounty hunters for patient referrals, so did their competitors. He said that the company had halted the practice on September 1, when it became illegal in Texas. "I am personally sick and tired of being bled to death by innuendo," Eamer said. He compared himself to Supreme Court Justice Clarence Thomas, the subject of brutal confirmation hearings over sexual harassment charges, except, he said, "I don't have an official accuser."

Actually, innuendo was not what NME was being hit with—the charges starting to spill out were sharp, direct and specific. And among the "official accusers" was the state attorney general, Dan Morales—who, Eamer later scoffed, "hasn't got the vaguest idea of what he's doing." Eamer mused about Morales's "political ambitions" and accused him of "not exercising good faith." In an interview in the *Dallas News*, the combative Eamer suggested that since NME's thirteen Texas hospitals had accounted for only $3.1 million of the $10 million in claims to the state Crime Victims Compensation Fund, "I guess that means we're only 31 percent of the problem, and the other 69 percent belongs to someone else."

Eamer, insisting that "there are no overcharges, no kidnapings," threatened to sue Morales for having "a vendetta against people giving psychiatric care." He told the *Houston Chronicle*, "I think they picked on us because we're the largest psychiatric hospital chain. I intend to do something about it. I'm mad and I feel extraordinarily belligerent."

This stance, while perhaps reassuring to NME's top officials and

45,000 employees, did little to calm the stock market, where investors fretted over an accelerating decline in occupancy rates at NME hospitals in Texas as the allegations swirled. Nor did it dissuade state investigators. Stunned by what he had been hearing from former patients, for example, Moncrief marveled at "what was crawling out from under the rocks every time we lift one up." He referred to the psychiatric-hospital problem as "one of the largest scandals in this state's history."

The state attorney general also had come to believe that the abuses were not isolated cases. Indeed, Morales contended, the very object of for-profit psychiatric hospitals' existence was "to gain access to public and private insurance funds." He said he had begun hearing from prosecutors in other states and estimated that at least ten other investigations into the psychiatric-hospital industry had begun outside Texas.

Psychiatric-hospital-industry spokesmen insisted that the intensifying criticisms were overshadowing the crucial need for their services. On October 16, when a berserk gunman opened fire in a restaurant in Kileen, Texas, killing twenty-four people, including himself, and wounding others, NME moved to underscore the point.

On October 27, its psychiatric division, PIA, took out newspaper ads headlined, "A Dose of Reality from PIA" and saying that the company had been "unfairly criticized for allegedly putting profits ahead of patients." In the past year, PIA said, its hospitals had treated more than 13,000 patients with psychiatric illnesses and substance-abuse problems in Texas. The ads pointed to the Kileen massacre as "a graphic reminder of the dramatic need for our services," and added, "We strongly resent allegations by the Attorney General's office that PIA 'kidnapped' Texans."

As new hearings were set to open in the fall, NME delivered a written statement to be read into the committee's record: "PIA has been hurt by these allegations. Our reputation has been damaged unfairly. We have been hurt, in terms of lost patients, but also because professionals and agencies who have referred patients to us in the past are now afraid to do so."

NME said it was "appalled by some of these allegations and we, like you, have been taking action" to investigate the charges and "provide recommendations." Said the statement: "It is not now and never has been the policy of PIA or NME to pay for the referral of prospective patients."

The statement called attention to the fact that many of the former patients making allegations against psychiatric hospitals were, of course, people who had problems. "It is unfortunate in psychiatric care that not all patients are satisfied. Not all are cured," NME pointed out.

Marketing concerns were not neglected, even in a letter to an investigating committee. The statement warned of the dangers of denial of mental disorders and the damage posed by increasing fears about the "still-pervasive stigma of mental illness." It exhorted the senators to remain objective for the sake, at least, of the children. "For example, the U.S. Office of Technology Assessment estimates that only 20 percent of the some 12 million children nationally in need of mental health services are receiving them."

On October 25, the first in a statewide series of formal hearings opened before a standing-room-only crowd of more than 250, packed into an auditorium and spilling out into hallways at the University of Texas campus in Arlington. Over several days, sixty witnesses testified—carpenters, truck drivers, nurses, lawyers, secretaries, teenagers working summer jobs—all with the same basic story of experiencing or witnessing abuses by psychiatric hospitals whose administrators exhibited an overpowering interest in milking insurance benefits. Additional hearings were already scheduled for San Antonio and Houston. The sessions took on an air of political rally. Often a victim's testimony was applauded; many witnesses, who had been frightened about going public, said that they were relieved to realize that they were not alone. On the other hand, some psychiatric hospitals encouraged staff members to attend to lend support to their employers. Willowbrook Hospital administrator Tom Edgar, for one, wrote to employees, affiliated doctors, and subcontractors, asking them to "openly show your support" by attending the hearings, speaking in the hospital's defense, and wearing a blue ribbon, which he enclosed with his letter.

Listening to reports about the standard use of "rage reduction therapy" and "chair therapy," Moncrief said: "It boggles the mind. I'm not a doctor, but good gosh, Gertie, this is absurd."

One of the numerous professionals who testified was Charles Arnold, the San Antonio psychiatrist who had blown the whistle on recruiting. He said that "a large number of psychiatrists, psychologists, counselors, therapists and psychiatric hospitals have betrayed the public trust and have, in effect, sold their souls" to profit from "the over-utilization of psychiatric hospitals and the excessive provision of psychiatric care."

At hearings that had reconvened in San Antonio in mid-November, Senator Harris showed Dr. Arnold a handful of hospital bills for several patients, calling them "obvious, flagrant bills where it was physically impossible for the patient to have digested the amount of medication that they allegedly were put on." Arnold frowned, studying the items listing drugs billed, suggesting that the patient who took all of those drugs at the times indicated would be dead. "I hope this is a typographical error," he said. "If not, this is criminal." By the time of the hearings, six years after he first began getting disgusted by what he had seen, Arnold said he was planning an early retirement.

Sheldon Silk, a private-practice psychologist and former regional vice president for a group of private psychiatric hospitals in the Midwest, told the hearing bluntly: "Texas has a long-standing history of having among the highest reimbursement rates for psychiatric and substance-abuse care in the entire country, very long lengths of stay, and flagrant practices of infiltrating schools and court systems with paid staff to offer free services."

Silk added, "During my career I have personally witnessed innumerable situations involving payment or bounties for referral of patients to hospitals; quota systems for employees to maintain referral rates and census figures or face termination; physicians using lesser trained professionals to deliver patient care and billing as if the M.D. had actually delivered the care; administrators forging documents and constructing false and bogus documentation to escape from closer scrutiny. I have seen treatment plans and various medical record components altered or redone to increase reimbursement from payers. As a professional, I endured and suffered tremendous indignities in my efforts to maintain a reasonable level of quality patient care while the corporation demanded higher financial returns. . . ."

Another witness, Wallace Thomas, said that he had responded to an advertising brochure and taken his eight-year-old daughter with "behavioral problems" to a free evaluation session at NME's Arbor Creek Hospital near Dallas. There, after filling out a detailed evaluation sheet, Thomas was asked details of his insurance. Once the "outreach officer" saw his insurance card, she suggested that not only the child, but the *entire family*—Thomas, his wife, and all three of their children—be hospitalized. "If one of you needs inpatient care, you all need it," the hospital evaluator told him. The family was hospitalized together for three days, before the Thomases, having consulting with their insurance company, checked themselves out.

A counselor recounted how recruiters deliberately got wavering potential patients drunk to persuade them to sign in for alcohol treatment. A former patient showed a bill listing thirty-eight different drugs prescribed in one day.

Listening to these kinds of allegations while attending the hearings at one session at Rice University, Texas governor Ann Richards, who had described herself as a recovering alcoholic, walked out in a fury, and ran into an unlucky official from a state mental-health agency in the hallway. "You better get your act together," she barked at the quaking bureaucrat, "and you better get it together before these hearings end!"

On November 18, a week after the stock bumped bottom at its lowest price in a year, NME's senior executive vice president John C. Bedrosian, one of the company's founders, took a more conciliatory stance. In a three-page letter to Moncrief, he allowed that some mistakes may have been made: "I'm not writing to tell you that PIA is perfect. I know we have done some things operationally in Texas I'm not proud of." Bedrosian reported that the company had canceled sixty-three business contracts that "do not meet the requirements" of the September 1 state law prohibiting the paying of bounties for patient referrals.

NME's reputation "for the highest ethical and legal principles," he wrote, "only deepens the shame we feel over the present problems in Texas." Still, Bedrosian seemed to suggest to the politicians, consider the source: The "individual patient cases" being revealed in testimony, as well as the "irresponsible reporting" in the Texas press, had presented "just one side of very complex stories"— stories, he noted, being told by psychiatric patients who had been "entrusted to our care. . . . I urge the committee to take the necessary steps to examine the medical records of patients who come before you."

On November 20, NME executives, aware of laws requiring publicly traded corporations to disclose bad news to investors in a timely manner, informed stock analysts at a meeting in Phoenix that earnings at the psychiatric hospitals would be well below previous estimates. Bedrosian blamed "unsubstantiated allegations of wrongdoing" for reducing patient days at the hospitals in Texas. The announcement precipitated heavy selling of the stock, which was again the most actively traded on the New York Stock Exchange.

The next day, hours after state mental-health licensing inspectors arrived for a surprise inspection of Psychiatric Institute of Fort Worth to examine records and interview staff members about the treatment of twelve patients whose families had alleged abuses, the hospital's administrator for the past five months, David Brockett, abruptly resigned.

On November 25, the Texas attorney general's office said it had expanded the investigation to include allegations against Charter, CPC, and HCA, including charges that recruiters for psychiatric hospitals had been "worming their way into school districts."

The story found its way onto national television again in December, when Senator Zaffirini was interviewed on the *Oprah Winfrey Show* and discussed the allegations against the Psychiatric Institute of Fort Worth. Ironically, a thirty-eight-year-old Fort Worth man, a retired Air Force technician, happened to be watching the show from a Psychiatric Institute of Fort Worth hospital bed, where he had been confined against his will since the day before. His estranged wife had had him committed, alleging in a warrant for emergency detention that he suffered from mood swings and was a danger to himself. Protesting his apprehension, the man was told he was in "denial," he told the *Dallas Morning News*, and informed that the only way he could get out soon was to voluntarily commit himself for an evaluation. The man's sister, watching *Oprah* in Chicago and aware of her brother's hospitalization, flew to Texas and got him out.

By the time the new year came around, the publicity in Texas had taken its toll. Eamer was now conceding that mistakes had been made, that some NME hospitals had engaged in "overly aggressive marketing." He told the *Houston Chronicle*, "I think we put too much pressure on our employees in the tough marketplace in Texas." But, he added, "I don't think we did anything different than any of the other chains."

Eamer maintained that he was "flabbergasted" by the revelations about the company he helped to found: "It's like picking up the newspaper and reading that your wife has left with someone."

CHAPTER SIXTEEN

....

THE MENTAL-HOSPITAL SCANDALS HAD THEIR ORIGINS, AS SO
many American scandals do, in an atmosphere of optimism and
good intentions—in this case, Lyndon Johnson's War on Poverty
of the middle 1960s.

The idea was laudable—to guarantee medical care, chiefly hospital treatment, for the poor and for those over the age of sixty-
five. Old people use general hospitals at a rate four times higher
than the rest of the population. The programs devised to subsidize
that care—federally funded Medicare for the elderly and federal-
and-state-funded Medicaid for the poor—also proved to be a financial bonanza for what was rapidly becoming known as the
"health-care industry," since they guaranteed reimbursements at
a fixed percentage above costs.

Besides providing a safety cushion for millions of Americans,
these programs created, virtually overnight, a thriving, ravenous
corporate hospital industry. The industry grew on financial rewards
and tax incentives that encouraged expansion, acquisition of competitors, and ambitious new construction. Now beholden to Wall
Street's demands for higher profits every quarter, the typical U.S.
hospital could no longer get along year in and year out providing
a reasonable level of community service and paying its bills. Like

the savings-and-loan, the hospital became a virtually unregulated, investor-driven enterprise, fiscal eye fixed coldly on the quarterly earnings report, one more profit center hustling in the sweeping corporatization of American health care, which had become the nation's second-largest industry, after defense. Before long, hospitals were managing to take in forty cents out of every health-care dollar spent in America.

Not coincidentally, overall U.S. health-care spending went up sharply, with widely expanding employee health-insurance benefits taking their place in the revenue stream beside the huge federal insurance programs. Indeed, the explosion in U.S. health-care spending over the past thirty years has paralleled the rapid expansion of payment by these third-party payers (from 51 percent of total U.S. health-care spending in 1960 to over 80 percent in 1993). In 1965, when Medicare and Medicaid were enacted, the total U.S. health-care bill was $65 billion; in 1993, it would be $939 billion.

From this wholesale revamping of American health-care economics emerged giant national hospital corporations such as Humana, American Medical International, Hospital Corporation of America, and National Medical Enterprises, all growing fast and changing the face of U.S. hospitals. By 1985, 39 percent of all U.S. community hospitals were owned by a multi-unit organization, including big national chains and smaller regional groups, profit or nonprofit. By 1990, nearly half were. Fat with government and insurance-company largesse, the tightly managed, aggressively marketed hospital companies became darlings of Wall Street.

By the Reagan administration, with deregulation a national byword, Medicare money had become the chief source of revenue for most hospitals and many American doctors. With the economy thriving and the postwar baby-boom population aging toward its prime hospital-using years, it looked as if this goose would never stop laying golden eggs.

But in 1983, in what was presented as a correction to take control

of soaring medical costs, Congress passed a federal reimbursement system for Medicare based on "DRGs"—diagnostic-related
groups—which fixed standard fees for specific treatments. The
DRG system is famously complex and annoying to hospitals and
physicians. There are almost five hundred separate DRGs, under
which hospitals are paid a certain fee for a specific treatment,
usually regardless of how long the patient is hospitalized. While
the fact was little noted in 1983, the corporate hospital chains and
medical associations had aggressively lobbied for DRGs—indeed,
had designed the key elements of the system. Overwhelmingly,
the new system rewarded efficiently managed chain hospitals, encouraging them to concentrate on the most profitable treatments
(and patients) and to turn over beds as rapidly as possible—which
meant that advertising and marketing became increasingly important as a way to bring in customers. By the end of the decade, U.S.
hospitals were spending an aggregate $1.5 billion on advertising
and marketing, according to industry estimates.

As it was designed, the system favored chain hospitals with their
corporate cost-efficiency and high debt-to-asset ratios. It encouraged them to build new facilities and add expensive new technol-
ogies to market services and create new ones. The system also had
the effect of impoverishing competing nonprofit or free-standing
for-profit general hospitals, hundreds of which simply sold out to
chains. By the end of the decade, one out of four U.S. hospitals
would be owned by a national corporate chain.

This shift profoundly changed U.S. health care. For the first
time, hospital patients were classified primarily according to their
potential for producing revenue. Hospital executive suites now
bustled with a new breed of professional: the marketing expert,
an executive whose background was often not in health care but
in such fields as hotel management, fast-food franchising, and
advertising.

But as carefully as it was designed by the hospital industry and
a compliant federal government, the DRG system turned out not

to be the blessing the hospital chains had expected. In 1985, as part of the Gramm-Rudman budget deficit reduction act, a cantankerous Congress made annual DRG rate increases part of the budget process, which curtailed their anticipated growth rates. Meanwhile, private insurance companies took the opportunity to limit reimbursements correspondingly, while raising deductibles and imposing new constraints such as pre-admission reviews for hospitalization. And state governments, reeling from across-the-board cutbacks in federal funding, began slashing at their own contributions to Medicaid. At the same time, thanks to competition from medical clinics, outpatient treatment was growing rapidly; lengths of hospital stays declined sharply. The climate for full-service medical hospitals had changed almost overnight. By 1985, hospital admissions were off 10 percent from their peak in 1981.

In their zeal to expand in the 1970s and early 1980s the corporate-hospital high-fliers had failed to heed warnings that the acute-care-hospital business was becoming precariously overbuilt and perilously deep in debt. Ironically, the champions of free enterprise in health care had received what they asked for: unfettered competition, which left the market glutted just as the money slowed down.

Hit by enormous declines in hospital utilization rates, the market reacted naturally. In 1985, Wall Street's health-care sector reverberated with a resounding crash in hospital stock prices.

As the dust settled, some medical companies had reason to be pleased by their foresight. During the Recovery Era, when public attitudes became more conditioned to accept intervention in personal behavior, some of these medical companies had begun investing heavily in a totally different segment of the health-care business: psychiatric hospitals. Thanks to incessant marketing and wily lobbying, health insurers were persuaded—and in many cases legally required—to provide coverage for a whole range of psychiatric and addiction treatments. And ironically (since psychiatric treatment defies standard evaluation in a way that, say, heart sur-

gery or obstetrics does not), psychiatric hospitals depending on
third-party reimbursement from Medicare, Medicaid, and employer health benefits managed to remain exempt from the now-
hated DRG controls. The American Psychiatric Association, arms
linked with the National Association of Private Psychiatric Hospitals, had led the intensive lobbying effort that ensured that
outcome.

By the end of 1985, there were nearly 250 private psychiatric
hospitals in the United States—and another 150 under construction, many of them being built in states such as Texas and California,
where lobbying had successfully abolished certificate-of-need laws.

By the end of the decade, four psychiatric-hospital corporations
controlled about 80 percent of the industry. The rest of the market
was divvied up by a scattering of mostly regional corporations,
some owned by investors affiliated with religious organizations.
Additionally, general hospitals offered competition with more limited, but also heavily marketed, psychiatric programs. In the brief
life span of the psychiatric-hospital industry, the focus in treatment
was decisively on customers with insurance. Publicly funded care
for indigents languished: From 1970 to 1986, the number of psychiatric beds available in state and county mental hospitals fell from
more than 400,000 to fewer than 120,000.

Of the Big Four psychiatric-hospital firms, National Medical Enterprises ultimately found itself in the most trouble in Texas and
elsewhere. By 1993, NME and the ethical practices of its psychiatric hospitals were the subject of fourteen separate federal and
state investigations, according to *The Wall Street Journal*. Based
in Santa Monica, California, NME owned seventy-six psychiatric
hospitals in twenty-four states at the end of 1991. Only ten years
before, the company had owned three psychiatric hospitals. The
1980s had been quite a run.

NME's founders—Richard Eamer, Leonard Cohen, and John Bedrosian—were lawyer-businessmen from southern California. In

the late sixties, Eamer represented a small group of regional hospitals as a tax attorney. Infused with the entrepreneurial spirit, he had admired the growth of the first major for-profit hospital chain, American Medical International, another California enterprise. (AMI's founder, Uranus J. "Bob" Appel, had started with a medical laboratory doing work for various hospitals. With experience in the hotel and restaurant businss, Appel moved into hospitals, beginning in the 1960s with a small facility in Los Angeles and expanding rapidly, first northward into central California and then into Texas and elsewhere.)

With Medicare and Medicaid money revolutionizing health care and opening it to investors who thought big, Eamer formed an investment group of physicians and lawyers who bought control of four general hospitals and three convalescent homes. In 1969, National Medical Enterprises went public with a $25.5 million stock offering that pointed out the vast profit potential from new governmental insurance reimbursements. By 1971, Eamer had become a well-known proselytizer for investor-owned hospital chains, which, he said in the trade magazine *Modern Hospital*, offered the allure of labor expenses 20 to 25 percent lower than those of non-profit hospitals in California, which typically had union workforces and large staffs.

In April 1982, NME moved boldly and presciently into the psychiatric-hospital business, paying $100 million to acquire a thriving Washington, D.C.–based company called Psychiatric Institutes of America, which then owned twenty-one psychiatric hospitals and four addiction-treatment centers in thirteen states.

Correctly forecasting the imminent boom in inpatient psychiatric care, Eamer enthusiastically told stockholders in the annual report: "The private psychiatric hospital industry is growing at an average annual rate of 26 percent as rehabiliatation continues to shift from government institutions to the community and private sector." One especially attractive aspect of PIA was its revenue source: Almost 90 percent of the patient revenue came from reimbursements by private insurers, an unheard-of percentage in the hospital industry, which depended largely on government reimbursements.

PIA was an innovator in the profit-making psychiatric-hospital industry. The company was started in 1969 in Washington, D.C., by Edward S. Fleming, a wealthy psychiatrist known to his colleagues at George Washington University Medical School as a financial wizard with a flair for creative marketing. Fleming and seven psychiatrists who came in with him as partners opened Washington's first for-profit psychiatric hospital. The key to the hospital's spectacular economic success was a philosophy of treatment called "milieu therapy" that had been pioneered by so-called child guidance clinics after the First World War and later adopted by the Menninger Clinic.

The idea was simple. If mental health was defined as an active state of social and emotional well-being, it followed that treatment of mental disorders needed to be aggressive and comprehensive. If (as critics of the state asylum "snake pits" in the forties and fifties had clearly revealed) the old-style mental institution had been part of the cause of mental illness itself, a new-style treatment facility should itself be part of the cure. Thus a psychiatric hospital's ethos—not only care from physicians and nurses, but interpersonal relationships, routine discussions with staff, recreational services and facilities, and even such details as the color of the walls and the selection of music piped into rooms—could be considered essential components of the treatment process.

In milieu therapy, "the total environment is part of the treatment," according to *The Psychiatric Therapies*, a standard psychiatric textbook published in 1984 by the American Psychiatric Association. In such an environment, a nonmedical staff worker who leads a group in dance steps, painting, or music appreciation is by definition a therapist. For example, *The Psychiatric Therapies* describes dance therapy, art therapy, and drama therapy as well-established "psychotherapeutic" techniques.

While the idea of an all-encompassing milieu therapy has obvious therapeutic and humane virtues, it has extraordinary economic ones, too, in a for-profit setting. Once the philosophy of milieu therapy was firmly established, and accepted by insurance payers, a psychiatric hospital was able to better justify extended patient stays, and to increase its daily rate to cover not only room and board, but a wide range of other routine services, seven days a week. Moreover, since it shared some historical roots with well-established and much-admired principles of nursery-school organization devised by the Italian psychiatrist Dr. Maria Montessori, milieu therapy was particularly conducive to justifying the psychiatric hospitalization of children and adolescents, who would soon become the strongest growth segment of the for-profit psychiatric industry.

Milieu therapy also emphasized the involvement of families and community social workers. At PIA, terms like "crisis intervention" and "co-dependency" were in use long before they became fashionable later in the Recovery Era.

Within a few years of its founding, PIA, despite daily room charges that compared with those at full-service acute-care hospitals in Wasington, was posting 90 percent occupancy rates, the highest in the for-profit hospital business.

NME's first initiative after acquiring this cash cow was to cut staff and housekeeping costs while putting more money into the new subsidiary's already aggressive marketing program. Within a year, thrilled by PIA's robust earnings, Eamer repositioned his company for a bold new future in which psychiatric care would be an integral part of medical care. He told investors that "at least 50 percent, and possibly as much as 80 percent, of all visits to physicians" could be traced to psychological or substance-abuse problems. Eamer foresaw astonishing growth in the psychiatric hospital industry generally, predicting that "at least 50,000 additional psychiatric beds" would be needed within two years.

Over the years, PIA's marketing acumen was widely admired and imitated in the burgeoning for-profit psychiatric hospital industry. As it expanded rapidly through the seventies, for example, PIA established a nonprofit foundation to devise "training programs" for clergymen, teachers, drug abuse counselors, and nurses.

In its early years, PIA had numerous critics among its competitors within the mental-health establishment of Washington and its Virginia and Maryland suburbs. One early opponent in Montgomery County, Maryland, was Dr. William Clotworthy, Jr. Speaking at a county meeting in support of county nonprofit mental-health facilities who feared the PIA would skim the revenue-producing patients off the market, Dr. Clotworthy charged that PIA-affiliated psychiatrists hospitalized their patients too often and for too long "because insurance covers only inpatient-type hospital care." At the same public meeting, another opponent said of PIA: "The length of stay of patients tracks remarkably well with the duration of their insurance coverage." A PIA official responded that while the average length of stay was twenty-eight days, most policies at that time covered a full year of hospitalization.

Like other psychiatric-hospital companies, NME made giant strides in the mid-eighties, while reimbursement limits and other factors battered the general-hospital business. Although NME announced a fourth-quarter loss of $25 million in 1986 because of the downturn in its once-thriving general-hospital business, the company restructured itself to devote most of its energy—and a billion dollars—to building more psychiatric hospitals.

In 1984, NME had owned twenty-five psychiatric hospitals and five addiction-treatment centers. Eamer, by now referring to mental illness as a "commonplace ailment," regaled stockholders that year with medicalized psychiatry's visions of "expanding the scope of treatment to meet the specific needs of specialized disorders" and even foreseeing "inoculations" to "treat psychiatric disorders." In his annual letter to shareholders, he boasted of the company's "reputation for successful care of the 'treatment-resistant' patient," by establishing twenty-four-hour-a-day crisis-intervention services

to facilitate admissions and expanding psychiatric-hospital programs for children, assisted by a major advertising campaign. Soon
to come, Eamer said, were "specialized outreach programs, including holiday depression counseling, military family workshops,
and programs for the physically handicapped," as well as new "educational programs to schools and other groups," and outpatient
offices to provide follow-up care and to "identify new patients."
Eamer also cited the new 800-COCAINE hot line at the company's
Fair Oaks Hospital in New Jersey. Eamer credited it with "creating
a strong identity for the company's chemical abuse treatment
capabilities."

NME's psychiatric business took off. In 1987 alone, the company
opened ten new psychiatric hospitals, bringing its total to fifty-
seven; seven more were under construction. By 1989, the company
proclaimed, the psychiatric business was "the primary engine driving our growth." By 1991, NME had eight-six psychiatric hospitals,
which were contributing $1.74 billion in revenue (up 21 percent
in a year) and $320 million in operating profits. On paper, the
future looked stable; the number of psychiatric admissions was up
by a robust 46 percent over 1989, for example. But though the
number of people being admitted rose, the average length of time
they spent in the hospital was down to twenty-four days in 1991,
compared with thirty days in 1989. The contrast was striking.

Aggressive marketing—the type that came to light in Texas—
had been bringing those new patients into the hospital, and the
house of cards was about to fall.

When it did, the other three big national psychiatric hospital
corporations under investigation in Texas and elsewhere also began
tottering.

Unlike NME, which maintained about half of its business in
general medical hospitals, Charter Medical Corporation was up to
its teeth in psychiatric hospitals when the Texas troubles swept
over the industry. Charter ended up in bankruptcy.

Like NME, Charter, headquartered in Macon, Georgia, had

started out in the late sixties as a regional chain. Its founder, William A. Fickling, parlayed eight general hospitals, nursing homes, and a construction subsidiary into a fast-growing psychiatric chain, which he took into its second decade proclaiming an ambitious goal: "to become the nation's leader in psychiatric hospital care," care that would be provided not in the psychiatric wings of general hospitals but in the "total treatment environment" of free-standing mental hospitals. Fickling was talking about what his competitors at PIA called milieu therapy.

His goal was realized. During the furious growth of the eighties, Charter expanded from fourteen psychiatric hospitals with about a thousand beds to eighty-four psychiatric hospitals and 7,629 beds, in twenty-seven states.

As his company prospered, Fickling emerged as the leading corporate figure in the psychiatric industry. His influence was felt all over the mental-health field, from grassroots marketing to Congress. Fickling's annual letters to shareholders rang with denunciations of government regulation and calls for "market-oriented" solutions to the problem of providing health care. Cheering Ronald Reagan's election as President, he reminded shareholders: "The platform on which the Republican candidates ran so successfully said about health care: 'What ails American medicine is government meddling and the straitjacket of federal programs. The prescription for good health care is deregulation and an emphasis on consumer rights and patient choice.' "

Charter worked hard at deregulation, especially in challenging certificate-of-need laws. The company's 1982 annual report stated a goal "of identifying progressive communities whose growth indicates that the type of innovative psychiatric hospital services Charter Medical provides will be a positive factor in the area's progress." For Charter and others expanding into the psychiatric-care business, this meant the Sunbelt, where regulations were looser, politicians friendlier, and insurance benefits attractive.

The money flooded in as new hospitals opened up. Charter's

revenues were $228 million in 1981, up 41 percent in just a year. Profits were up 59 percent. The next year, Fickling told investors about "the most active psychiatric hospital construction program in our highly competitive industry." Charter, he said, had become "a world leader in psychiatric hospital care."

By 1984, a year after Congress revised Medicare reimbursement policies in a way that favored big psychiatric-hospital chains, Fickling said that Charter was looking to grow in such areas as "geriatric psychiatry," since it was widely proclaimed that the elderly were increasingly suffering from depression. Fickling's letter to shareholders that year extolled the growing opportunities for hospital psychiatry: "A recent landmark study by the National Institute of Mental Health indicated that the incidence of psychiatric disorders and serious substance abuse in the U.S. is considerably higher than previously thought. . . . The country's mental health needs are underserved."

By 1987, with 5,647 psychiatric beds, Charter's revenues exceeded $1 billion, and there was no end in sight. That year the company spent a total of $185 million on construction of psychiatric facilities and filed eighteen new certificate-of-need applications for psychiatric hospitals.

Then Fickling and a group of other senior executives suddenly took the company private in a $1.5 billion leveraged buyout. The greatest of 1980s financial ploys, leveraged buyouts were breathtaking deals, supported by mountains of debt and rosy expectations, in which a group of senior managers essentially purchased a company at an inflated price, using money raised by audacious Wall Street speculators. The money was expected to be repayable through the unending good fortune of the company.

Exuberant, Charter borrowed still another $100 million to continue building new psychiatric hospitals, planning to raise its total to more than a hundred. Now saddled with debt exceeding $1.6 billion, Charter, spending about $40 million a year just for advertising, embarked on its new life as a private company just as the insurers began to trim the sails of the psychiatric industry in the late eighties.

The situation deteriorated rapidly. In 1990, the U.S. Department of Health and Human Services began investigating allegations of fraud in Medicare and Medicaid billing by Charter psychiatric hospitals from 1987 to 1989. Charter ultimately settled the charges over $850,000 in claims, paying Medicare an additional $948,000 for such things as costs of the investigation.

The company then laid off 2,600 employees, shut down several hospitals, and stunned investors who had purchased its high-interest bonds during the buyout by announcing that it had lost $311.3 million that year. But if 1990 was a bad year for Charter, 1991 was horrible.

Early in 1991, as losses mounted and due dates for big debt payments loomed, as whispers of possible default and bankruptcy were being heard over lunch, it seemed things couldn't get worse. They did. William Fickling was walking through the airport in Macon, Georgia, when he was approached by James W. Conte, the bottom-line-oriented chairman of Community Psychiatric Centers. Aware that his larger competitor probably couldn't come up with the money to make its next debt payment to bondholders, Conte informed the unhappy Fickling that he wanted to talk.

When Fickling balked, Conte threatened to take his deal directly to Fickling's nervous bondholders: $1.1 billion, cash and stock, to acquire Charter, add its eighty-nine psychiatric hospitals to CPC's fifty, and garner over a third of the U.S. corporate psychiatric-hospital industry. Fickling maintained that CPC was trying to destabilize the industry and gain competitve information, but Conte ridiculed that. "I don't see that a company with a 35 percent profit margin needs to gain any competitive advantage from a company that can't pay its debts," he told a reporter.

Aghast, Fickling took Charter to bankruptcy court instead.

At the time he made his audacious offer to buy out Charter,

Conte himself headed a company that investors regarded as the best-managed in the psychiatric business. CPC's stock was flying high, up nearly 50 percent in six months, following eighty-seven consecutive quarters of ever-increasing earnings.

But by 1991 analysts were starting to worry about CPC, too. The company's continuing good fortune appeared to be buoyed mostly by aggressive marketing and price increases. While rigorous corporate cost-cutting had kept CPC's bottom line in good shape, some analysts, with one eye on the trouble in Texas, warned that the good times might be ending.

Stock market analysts who followed psychiatric hospital companies began advising clients that CPC stock might be overvalued early in 1991. They were worried about indications that CPC was depending on what looked like an unsteady source of future revenue—Canadian patients.

The *Los Angeles Times* quoted Calvin Dufore, a former CPC vice president who had been responsible for recruiting patients from Canada. He said that CPC hospitals were bringing down so many patients from Canada that he had negotiated volume discounts with several airlines. He said CPC recruiters even frequented Canadian Salavation Army shelters in wintertime to recruit patients by showing videotapes of California CPC hospitals and their sun-drenched locales.

For Conte, who had racked up annual earnings growths exceeding 15 percent for nineteen straight years, whose salary had soared to more than $8 million a year by the end of the 1980s, who had been named "CEO of the Decade" by *Financial World Magazine*, it was an unexpected lesson in humility.

CPC had been one of the earliest corporate players in the psychiatric business. Conte and a partner, Robert L. Green, founded the company in the early 1960s, as state hospitals were beginning to empty of patients. The men started with one psychiatric hospital, in Belmont, California, near San Francisco.

As they were for the industry in general, the eighties were years of fabulous growth for CPC. Revenue in 1979 had been about $44 million; by 1982, when CPC owned nineteen psychiatric hospitals, annual revenue had shot up to $121 million. If NME had once boasted of its reputation as "Mr. Clean," CPC could say that it was "Mr. Lean." The company's byword was "efficiency"; it considered its operations to be the lowest-cost in the industry, but its rapid growth was also aided by aggressive establishment of relationships with local private-practice psychiatrists.

Like its competitors, in 1986 the company was poised for its biggest growth spurt ever. CPC announced plans to double its bed capacity—to nearly 4,500—in a two-year, $220 million construction spree. Encouraged by states that had dropped their certificate-of-need laws, CPC planned to open three new hospitals in Utah and Kansas that year, and ten in California and Texas in the next two years. By 1988, with annual revenue at $478.2 million, CPC happily told shareholders that admissions to its psychiatric hospitals were up 22 percent over 1987, thanks to stepped-up marketing and "crisis-intervention" programs. In words that would resonate with irony three years later, when the company needed to defend itself against accusations of unethical marketing, CPC founders Green and Conte, now the company's chairman and president, crowed in their 1988 letter to stockholders: "Over 60 percent of referrals to our hospitals now originate in the community, without the initial involvement of a psychiatrist." Besides referrals from clerics, teachers and school counselors, the courts, the police, and employee-assistance programs, the letter credited "the emergency wards of general hospitals" with the boost in psychiatric admissions. With the average length of stay now down to twenty-three days in the middle of the energetic construction program, however, it was clear that the pressure was on for still more admissions.

Two years later, Conte, now chairman, adopted an almost combative tone in his letter to shareholders. Brushing off the now-glaring publicity about "alleged problems" in the psychiatric-hospital industry, Conte asserted that the business was in a "shake-out period" that offered "significant opportunities."

In September 1991, Conte's retirement plans were put on hold after CPC announced that its now twenty-two-year-long string of consistently growing annual profits had come decisively to an end. There was a 98 percent drop in third-quarter profits. The fourth quarter was worse: The company took $16 million in charges against earnings to account for uncollected bills, including $7 million in claims for Canadian patients that had been rejected by the Ontario government. Announcing a loss of $3 million, CPC laid part of the blame on the fallout from the initial stages of the Texas investigations. On October 24, CPC stock fell $1.50 a share in heavy trading, to close at $12.875 on the New York Stock Exchange. Less than six months earlier, the stock had been at $40 a share.

The last of the Big Four, Hospital Corporation of America, was the only one founded by a physician. Perhaps as a result, HCA kept one foot firmly planted in the general-hospital business, and was less threatened when the psychiatric hospital business unexpectedly hit a wall in Texas.

HCA had been founded in 1965, when Thomas F. Frist, a Nashville cardiologist, opened a fifty-bed facility, Parkview Memorial Hospital. Fascinated by the possibilities of applying marketing principles to medical care, Frist had been one of the first medical entrepreneurs to see the opportunities for promoting recent revolutionary technological advances in cardiac treatment.

In 1968, to raise money and expand in the new medical era created by Medicare and Medicaid reimbursements, Frist teamed up with a former patient, Jack C. Massey, the marketing genius responsible for the rapid national growth of the Kentucky Fried Chicken chain. What had worked for fast-food chicken could work as well for medicine, Massey and Frist decided.

The company saw opportunities in psychiatric care in the

eighties; it acquired twenty-two psychiatric hospitals in 1981, with immediate profitable results. However, Frist, HCA's chairman, insisted that the company remain primarily a general-hospital enterprise, with the psychiatric business as a sideline. In 1985, HCA sent the first shock waves through the overconfident and newly overbuilt general-hospital industry, announcing its first bad earnings news. Wall Street reacted; as the bad news spread, the paper value of all publicly traded hospital companies dropped by $1.5 billion. But the Frists, like executives of the other major companies in the psychiatry business, could take satisfaction in their foresight. By the end of 1985, HCA owned forty psychiatric hospitals; revenues were up 45 percent, to $335 million.

Frist's son, Thomas Junior, a surgeon, became chairman in 1987 and moved HCA more forcefully into psychiatric care, concentrating on Sunbelt states, where he cited as his model for growth another franchise chain: Holiday Inn.

Early in 1987, with another eleven psychiatric hospitals under construction, HCA sold off 104 of its 196 general hospitals for $2.1 billion to an employee stock-ownership plan, in which it retained a significant ownership stake. In 1989, HCA, now with fifty-two psychiatric hospitals, followed the trend and went private, in a $5.1 *billion* leveraged buyout.

By 1990, HCA also found itself saddled with over $4 billion in debt, reporting an annual loss of $18.3 million, with a debt payment of $227 million coming due the next year. The company had been hoping to raise cash by selling its psychiatric hospitals for about $1.25 billion, but at about this time Senator Moncrief banged down the gavel again in Texas.

CHAPTER SEVENTEEN

....

Moncrief held up a memo dated December 23, 1991, more than three months after legislators in Texas had hastily passed a law making it illegal to pay bonuses and bounties for referring psychiatric patients to a hospital. The memo, under the letterhead "CPC Oak Bend Hospital, Fort Worth," described new admissions procedures at the hospital. "It's the following comment that concerns me," Moncrief said ruefully, turning a page. "It says, and I quote—it's in bold type—'You will receive credit for referrals to Oak Bend Hospital using the new method. Our intake staff will coordinate this tabulation.'" He put down the memo and peered at Loren B. Shook, the company's president. "Do you know what that means?"

Shook said he was not familiar with the document, but that he'd check into it.

"Well, you can see my reason for concern," Moncrief went on, "especially given the date . . . that's a pretty recent document. It's less than a month ago."

Shook said he doubted that the memo meant that staff psychiatrists and other employees were being offered bonuses for patient admissions. "I know we are not paying physicians."

"But it says, 'You *will receive credit*,'" Moncrief insisted.

257

"Credit," Shook replied tentatively. "That means you'll be counted [but] we do not pay them in any way for their admissions. That just simply means that patients being admitted will be credited to them with regard to statistically counting up how many patients Dr. X admitted to Oak Bend Hospital. . . . That's simply a business need for us to know is Dr. X no longer using our hospital, and if so, why. . . . We may find out that something was mishandled in some way with the treatment of that patient . . . so we've got to address that. . . . It's a very legitimate process."

The men who ran the psychiatric industry had been wrong when they told worried analysts and employees that the problems in Texas were local, isolated, and contained. As far as Moncrief and his colleagues were concerned, the problems were systemic, and national—perhaps international—in scope. The matter was not going to end in Texas.

By the end of 1991, even the normally docile health-care-industry trade publications were trumpeting the scandal with headlines and stories quoting people criticizing psychiatry with the kind of contempt that hadn't been heard in fifty years. The scandal was the main story in the December 1991 *Psychiatric Times*, the profession's official publication, which reported that five states were now actively investigating charges that corporate psychiatric hospitals engaged in kidnaping and "paying bounties to teachers, probation officers and psychiatrists," as well as "holding patients until their insurance . . . is depleted and then dumping them." Still, the trade journal worked up its greatest lamentations in the form of a sermon to the congregation: "The real losers in this battle, however, are the patients. Currently, only about half of those diagnosed with mental illness are getting care, according to an economist with the National Institute of Mental Health."

Industry executives like Shook made it a point to caution investigators that—while of course it was clear they meant well in exposing the anecdotal abuses—condemning the system itself would frighten away millions of Americans who required psychiatric treatment. "They're not going out and getting the care because of the publicity they've heard," Shook warned.

Shook firmly denied that the company paid bonuses to CPC employees for bringing in new patients. He also defended the aggressiveness with which CPC responded to disasters and tragedies—as in cases, he said, where schoolchildren are murdered. "It is common for CPC hospitals and other psychiatric hospitals in the state to make available free counseling services to the students and teachers when a tragedy occurs . . . ," he said.

But Moncrief pressed Shook on the "Canadian connection for patients, which I understand that CPC was involved in . . . opening offices in Canada for recruitment of patients. It's my understanding that at that time, the Canadian government was paying, through their health care, approximately 75 percent of the cost, the remaining 25 percent to be collected from the patients themselves. You were involved in that process, is that correct?"

"I'm aware of that, Senator. Yes."

At NME, the company receiving most of the bad press, the resolve to stonewall had begun to crumble before the end of 1991, as executives tried to put as much distance as they could between the corporate staff in Santa Monica and the once-prized psychiatric operation in Washington, which had been generating most of the company's profits.

"We had a loose rein on the people running the organization," Eamer explained. He did not mention that Zober, the NME senior vice president who ran the psychiatric hospitals, was also a member of NME's board of directors.

In mid-December, after placing Zober on paid leave and firing four other top executives, NME announced that it would eliminate the PIA name from its psychiatric operations. Plans were hastily made to relocate fifty executives in the psychiatric operation from Washington to corporate headquarters in Santa Monica. There, they reported to NME's newly hired chief medical director and senior vice president for psychiatric operations, John P. Docherty, M.D. Docherty, a former medical director of an NME psychiatric hospital in New Hampshire, was also the former medical director of PIA's "Depression Helpline" call-in service. Before joining NME in 1985, he had been chief of "psychosocial research" at the National Institute of Mental Health.

A more conciliatory Eamer acknowledged there had been "overly aggressive marketing" in the Texas hospitals. But, he insisted, his competitors were doing the same thing.

The scandal had saddened him personally, Eamer said. "We were chagrined, flabbergasted, angry, excited." The company's internal investigation, the results of which NME would not disclose, had identified a major perpetrator, "the Number One culprit," Eamer informed the *Houston Chronicle*. This was an ex-employee, whom Eamer declined to identify but who, he confided, "is now a major shogun or bigwig at one of our major competitors. He was instrumental in setting up these marketing means in our facilities."

But with admissions to NME's Texas hospitals down 30 percent in just a few months, the company finally realized that press releases were not working. Early in January, John C. Bedrosian and two other NME executives filed stiffly into a Senate hearing room in Austin.

Senator Chris Harris set the tone, gruffly declaring that he wanted to move his seat closer to the uncomfortable hospital tycoons. "If it pleases the Chair," Harris drawled, peering at them suspiciously as he dragged his chair nearer, "I would like to sit over here so I can eyeball them. I can't see the whites of their eyes from where I was." No less than his colleague Moncrief, who had served on a psychiatric hospital's community board, Harris had felt betrayed by the industry: He had been a prominent supporter of state legislation, avidly lobbied for by the psychiatric hospitals, that required Texas health insurers to provide coverage of inpatient treatment for substance abuse.

Warily, Bedrosian introduced himself: "I am senior executive vice president of National Medical Enterprises and am one of three founders of the company. NME is the parent company of the former Psychiatric Institutes of America, PIA, which is now our psychiatric division." Bedrosian, a lawyer by training, tried to put the best face on the situation by declaring his company's concern about the allegations and its determination to "find the right ways to improve what we all know is a vital service." Then he read from a statement:

> *National Medical Enterprises sincerely regrets what has happened here in Texas. Despite some recent lapses, our long-term history is that of a company with a social conscience, a company that sincerely cares about the people that we serve. The events of the past year have alarmed our management. We're well aware that the restoration of NME's reputation in this state will hinge on the extent to which we restore public confidence in our company.*

Bedrosian saw the problem as stemming from the rapid growth in psychiatric treatment during the 1980s, when PIA "expanded and acquired new facilities at a tremendous pace."

> *. . . In retrospect, we now realize this growth was a case of too much too soon. Also, conditions in the psychiatric field changed quickly during the eighties, and NME did not adapt quickly enough to these changes.*
> *We acknowledge that there have been problems in the psychiatric hospital industry, and that a number of employees and contractors, including some of ours, have engaged in overly aggressive and unethical practices because they placed profits too high on their list of priorities. Several months ago when these serious allegations first surfaced, we initiated an intensive review of our internal operations and identified areas where problems did exist. NME's senior management was highly*

*disturbed over many of the things we found in our review. As
a result of our in-house investigation, many of the people who
were in charge last year no longer have jobs with us. Others
have greatly different responsibilities.*

Of bounties, Bedrosian said: "We are following a strict construction of the law prohibiting bounties." However, he defended the
referral networks:

*We still conduct a variety of outreach and informational pro-
grams. People with psychiatric or substance abuse problems
need to know that they're not alone or unique, and that help is
available. This can be described as marketing our services, and
it's something any mental health care provider has to do. Again,
since this is the area where some of our people used poor judgment, we focused a great deal of attention on this aspect.*

Conceding little beyond, perhaps, overzealousness to serve the
public coupled with a lapse in oversight, Bedrosian said: "I realize
that no matter what we might say today, there will remain lingering
questions. . . . We have acknowledged that PIA did contribute to
the problem, and I've attempted today to describe what we're doing
to correct our internal deficiencies."

Accompanying Bedrosian was Robert Constantine, a forty-five-
year-old mental-health administrator and former PIA vice president appointed in late November to supervise the thirteen
embattled psychiatric hospitals in Texas. Constantine told the legislators that at NME hospitals "our admissions staff do not operate
under a quota system" and that "involuntary admissions and emergency detentions are done strictly in accordance with state law,
and with complete and appropriate documentation."

Frowning, Senator Zaffirini, who had favored giving the committee subpoena powers to force full cooperation from the corporations, noted Constantine's use of the present tense. "Are you

saying, that this is the history of your corporation and your institution? Or are you saying that these are the corrected measures which you have taken and that this will be the behavior in the future?"

"What I'm describing characterizes our operations as we speak," Constantine replied.

"You're not saying that this has been the history?"

"No, not in every case."

Constantine also sounded the theme that many of those criticizing corporate psychiatry's aggressive recruiting of patients could be in "denial" of mental disorders that sometimes are flushed out only through "intervention." Said Constantine, "The area of marketing is one that's gotten a lot of attention, and one where we've made major efforts. In the field of psychiatric and substance abuse care, denial is an everyday reality. Many patients who are hurting themselves with alcohol or drugs or through psychiatric problems simply don't accept the fact that they need help. We and other mental health professionals have to reach out to these people. A person with a broken leg knows he needs medical care—a person with a drug problem often doesn't. One way that we attempt to overcome denial is to try to educate people about the possible problems and inform them about their options for getting help."

To do this, he said, psychiatric hospitals need to maintain "personal contacts with physicians, teachers, judges, police, counselors and others whose work brings them into contact with those who need mental health or chemical dependency treatment. We talk to these people because we want to know what problems they are seeing, and we want to know what we can do to respond to these problems. There is nothing sinister or underhanded in these conversations and these contacts. We do encourage, in fact, these people to refer patients to us if they believe they need the level of care that we provide.

"We have made certain that decisions are made by physicians and based on patients' medical needs. . . . Patients are not kept in our hospitals until their insurance runs out. . . . It's important to understand, however, that insurance is a factor in psychiatric and substance abuse care, just as it is in all types of health care. . . . The goal is to meet our patients' needs within the framework of insurance benefits."

Senator Moncrief had perked up with the talk of consumer-oriented marketing. He interjected that he had been leafing through "some of the brochures that y'all used for the purpose of marketing."

He had in hand the infuriating "Books as Hooks" memo that had so irked him when he first started hearing about the trouble at psychiatric hospitals. Scowling, he read from it sarcastically, " 'Relapse and Recovery: "But I Don't *Feel* Sick" ' . . . 'Women in Recovery' . . . 'Books as Hooks.' " He had an assistant carry the brochure to Constantine and fixed him with a level stare. "Is this part of what you consider to be an ongoing marketing tool to increase census . . . and is it still being utilized?"

"Let me say a couple of things in response," Constantine said, marshaling his verb tenses once again. "First of all, my comments about our practices with regard to marketing and the clinical review of the content, as well as the legal review of the content, are a description of our current practices, not always our past practices. I'm not familiar with the document you're reading from, but my reaction to the words is that it reminds me of how loosely and sometimes inappropriately we've used words, with really the best of intentions."

Senator Harris didn't like the sound of this. "Did he go to law school?" he muttered. "I notice how he's been able to avoid answering your question."

"He has a Ph.D.," Senator Zaffirini said.

"Figures," grumbled Harris.

Constantine continued, "As I've said, we've used words loosely and inappropriately. But if you think about what's been said earlier with regard to marketing in educating the public, who are often denying that they've had problems, or not recognizing that they have problems, when you think about these kinds of books and their distribution in that context, they're doing precisely what we would like them to do. They're providing two things: One is help to the public in identifying if they have a problem, what it is. And the second is giving them some idea that they're probably not the only one that has that problem and that there are solutions to them—"

Moncrief snorted. "Doctor, now that book, 'Books as Hooks'— read that. Read some of the excerpts from that publication! That doesn't seem like that's helping anything but the institution itself to fill their beds!"

Uncomfortably, Constantine replied, "I would suggest that it is helping educate the public, but the word, the phrase 'Books as Hooks' is unfortunate—"

Bedrosian jumped in. "Don't answer that," he told his subordinate. "I'll be the lawyer. Don't answer that because you don't know what it says. It sounds terrible and probably is terrible. I haven't seen it either. I mean, I know the topic. When all this activity hit the press, that's when we in Los Angeles woke up to 'Hey, what's going on?' And we have to take responsibility for what's going on. I saw—I've never heard of this book, either, until right now."

Bedrosian conceded that NME hospitals had "problems" elsewhere besides Texas, but characterized them chiefly as public relations questions. "The problems that we've had in Florida and New Jersey in the press are different kinds of problems" from those in Texas, he said. "Rates of billings and things like that, primarily. They aren't marketing and aggressive marketing issues."

"What about Alabama, Louisiana and New York?" Zaffirini asked.

"New York? I don't know anything about New York."

Isolated instances aside, Bedrosian insisted, NME ultimately "woke up" to the problem it had with its marketing. Recently, he said, the PIA "Intake Manual," with its Golden Rules for keeping beds full, crossed his desk at corporate headquarters. "I read that Intake Manual for the first time, and it made me in a couple of areas sick to my stomach. And I'm not giving you lip service when I say that. I hated what I read, I was embarrassed by what I read in two or three instances in that manual, and obviously, we're revising it.

"Someone said to me, 'If PIA had been a manufacturing company in the last couple of years'—and I want to say the last couple of years because that's when the industry pressures began to increase, that's when marketing became more of an issue, that's when the payers began to become more aggressive in controlling what they wanted to pay, that's when it became harder to produce in what, up till then, had been an easy business to engage in. And I understand that because that's what happened to the acute hospital industry in this country until 1982 or '83—it was rapid growth, and growth covers a multitude of sins, and then it was shakeout. And we're in the shakeout mode in psychiatry, in terms of our industry."

Bedrosian found his train of thought, which was that treating mental illness is not as simple as making machine tools. "Someone said, if it was a manufacturing company, it would have been the best-run company in the country. The problem is that the medical component of the company . . . was changed. It was medically driven for many years. The doctors who created it, when we acquired it, it was medically driven—"

"Medically driven?" Moncrief inquired.

"It had been up until the last year, year and a half—"

"If it hasn't been medically driven the last couple of years, what has been the driving force?"

"The driving force has been to grow, grow, grow. I mean, because they grew for eight years, they thought they could keep growing forever," Bedrosian explained. "That's what it was."

"Growth for growth sake? Or growth for profit sake?

"The same thing, Senator."

266

Zaffirini came back to something that had been bothering her. Since the psychiatric business was so important to NME's profits, how could corporate executives not have known what was going on?

Bedrosian pointed out the complexity of managing a major national health-care corporation that had grown so rapidly. With so many general and psychiatric hospitals, he explained, "We had structured ourselves almost like a holding company. PIA had done well for years, and so we simply said, 'God bless you, keep going.'" Bedrosian reminded the senators that the psychiatric division was headquartered in Washington, D.C., "where the home office of PIA always was. It was there when they started the company—it will be moving to Los Angeles. We in Los Angeles are not that large a group that we are watching every single facility."

He continued, "In the old days, when we started our company in the sixties, up until the early seventies, the three of us who started the company went to every hospital board meeting and knew what was going on, and it worked well. But we just got too big."

Meanwhile, he insisted, "Not one instance that I can think of is there a clear-cut case where we really did everything, or did the things they said we did."

Bedrosian lamented that "the legalities constrain us" in defending against unfair allegations by former patients. "For the most part," he said, "these charges involve actions that can only be corroborated or refuted by looking at the files of individual patients. . . . We're prohibited by confidentiality laws from discussing the information contained in those files."

Bedrosian continued, "That frustrates me more than you will ever know. I've asked five different law firms, 'I want to talk to these cases publicly.' They won't let me! They said, 'You'll face a lawsuit if you do.'"

He gazed at the impassive faces of his interrogators on the senate panel. "I have to tell you that denial is a major factor in a lot of these cases, the denial that we talked about. We're talking about seventy people" [who had testified about abuses to date]. "Some of these people were ten years old. They're old stories. That doesn't mean they're to be ignored, but I don't want to give them the credence that they are the current state of the art, either. . . . The things we found [to be wrong], we've changed. We're a different company today than we were four months ago."

He characterized NME as a blameless victim, not only of disgruntled patients and ex-employees, but of the distance between PIA headquarters in Washington and corporate headquarters in California. "Okay. We didn't know about some of the conduct of the people who are no longer with us now," he said. "We didn't know about 'Books as Hooks,' or whatever. We didn't know about the language that we saw in some of our manuals. We didn't know about the aggressiveness of the environment in the marketplace. I have to admit that to you. But it was where we're structured to know. We had senior people who we were paying to do that for us."

Senator Zaffirini wanted to know about the marketing abuses.

"The marketing was a systemic thing, okay," Bedrosian admitted. "Not just PIA—the system." But he again returned to his assertion that the senior executives were in the dark on such abuses. "All of us, those who started the company, the senior structure, are in Los Angeles," he reiterated. PIA "was three thousand miles away."

Still, Zaffirini asked, why did he and other NME officials have to be subpoenaed to appear? "Why did you not come forth immediately?" she demanded.

"Because we thought we were wrongly maligned and accused of things that weren't true—because we knew the patient stories. A lot of them were not valid," Bedrosian said, adding: "When [the publicity] all started, we realized, 'Wait a minute—what's going on here? That's an awful lot of folks, and all of a sudden we're getting attacked from every which way.' The first thing we did was to put the gentleman in charge of this division [he was referring to Zober] on a leave of absence and start an internal investigation, because we didn't want to go out and say something immediately. We weren't prepared to talk to anybody. We didn't know what was going on, quite frankly, in some of the details of these allegations and the stories in the press and what have you. We didn't have the facts. We've been working very hard to find out what in Sam Hill is going on."

Bedrosian returned again to the industry's chief line of defense: "Whatever you all do, realize that there is an element of denial in health care. Please don't burden the provider industry by creating an easy opportunity for people to frankly harass us, and overuse statutes—"

This got Harris's dander up again. The senator said that, to prepare himself for Bedrosian's visit, he himself had recently telephoned a PIA crisis "help line" whose number he found in the phone book. "And I hope you're not the one who instructed the people to say the kind of things they say," he warned, wagging a finger.

"I'm not," Bedrosian said. "I would love to hear it—but not now."

Harris chuckled. "I understand you're trying to do something about it, but I promise you, your message has not gotten all the way down to the troops who are out there—"

"I know that—"

"—and are talking to these families who are hurting, who have genuine problems, who are desperate, and who are reaching out for help—"

"I know that."

"And do you know," Harris said sharply, "one of the first questions I got asked? How big is my insurance policy!"

EPILOGUE

....

ON AUGUST 26, 1993, EVENTS THAT HAD BEGUN MORE THAN TWO years earlier with the hospitalization of a teenaged boy from a San Antonio suburb culminated in a sad morning for employees of National Medical Enterprises, in hospitals all across the country. The company, which the *Wall Street Journal* had once referred to as the "Mr. Clean" of the psychiatric industry, was raided by more than five hundred FBI and other federal agents.

In Santa Monica, California, workers at NME's five-story headquarters watched forty law-enforcement officers search the building and cart away file cabinets and cartons of corporate documents. The same day, hundreds of other agents conducted raids against NME hospitals and regional offices in Texas, Colorado, Indiana, Arizona, Missouri, California, Washington, D.C., Florida, Virginia, Louisiana, Michigan, Georgia, Wisconsin, and Minnesota.

The raids were coordinated by the U.S. Justice Department, which had set up prosecution offices in a dozen U.S. cities to conduct a major federal investigation of health-care fraud, which is estimated to cost more than $70 billion a year. According to *The New York Times*, the action against NME was "part of an effort to prove that the company had participated in a national conspiracy to defraud patients and insurance companies."

Over two years, as allegations against NME and other hospital companies swirled out of Texas and spread nationally, NME had steadfastly maintained that instances of wrongdoing were isolated and confined to a few individual hospitals where administrators overreacted in the supercharged competitive atmosphere of the U.S. private psychiatric hospital industry during the late eighties and early nineties.

However, the *Wall Street Journal* reported in its account of the August 26 raids that "the government is said to believe those actions reflect a pattern of misconduct that spread from the giant hospital operator's executive suites, according to investigators and attorneys."

NME said it would cooperate with federal investigators. "We are hopeful that the records obtained today will help the government to put to rest many of its concerns, and in any event lead to a prompt resolution of the government's investigations," NME's general counsel, Scott Brown, said in a statement.

NME continued to refuse to comment on any of the estimated 130 individual lawsuits filed against its psychiatric hospitals by patients. The company maintained that it had been singled out unfairly in an industry where ambitious marketing was considered a virtue—until major insurance companies began feeling the pinch from corporations suddenly unwilling to continue paying the soaring costs of psychiatric and substance-addiction treatment.

In 1992, hoping to contain the damage in Texas, NME had agreed to a $7 million settlement of the lawsuit by the state attorney general. Under the terms, NME relinquished more than $3.4 million in claims on the crime victims fund, agreed to a number of reforms in marketing and admissions policies, and committed to providing additional charity care at its psychiatric hospitals. The company did not admit any wrongdoing. Robert Constantine, the head of NME's Texas psychiatric operations, said when the agreement was announced, "The problems we close the book on today arose in the last two years as Texas psychiatric hospitals became overbedded and went beyond the bounds of propriety."

But the book didn't stay closed for long. A month later, a group of major U.S. insurance companies filed a lawsuit charging NME with undertaking "a coordinated national scheme" to "secure the hospitalization of thousands of patients who did not need hospitalization." The complaint charged that NME "manipulated and/ or misstated diagnoses and treatment," and billed for services either not provided, or provided at "grossly inflated levels." According to the complaint, NME organized "vast referral networks" of psychiatrists and psychologists, independent agencies, school counselors, parole officers, emergency room nurses, telephone hotline workers, alcohol-abuse counselors, and employee-assistance-program officials to garner patients.

A second lawsuit against NME was filed two months later by two other insurance companies who said they paid "fraudulent claims" in what the complaint called "one of the most massive and pernicious health-care scandals of all time." This was followed in early 1993 by an additional suit by four more insurers. Together, the three suits identified more than $1 billion in claims paid to NME psychiatric hospitals.

NME responded that it had become a scapegoat for the insurance industry, which "has attempted to force hospitals and consumers to pay for the costs of medical services [that] the insurance companies are obligated to under their policies." Insurers, said NME, "are attempting to divert attention away from their responsibility for the increased cost of health insurance by placing the blame on physicians, hospitals and other health-care professionals and providers."

Complicating the situation somewhat was the fact that many insurance companies had financial interests in the psychiatric hospital industry. In 1991 a study by the Texas state insurance department found that eleven of the twenty-five U.S. health insurance companies had a total of about $1 billion invested in psychiatric hospitals and facilities. While the insurance industry pointed out that such investments represented only a small percentage of in- surers' portfolios, Senator Moncrief, for one, wasn't buying it. "If there ever was a conflict of interest, this is one," the Texas legislator said.

By 1993, however, NME was scrambling to repair the damage, as litigation piled up and the federal criminal investigation gathered steam. The three founders of the company, Eamer, Cohen, and Bedrosian, all were forced out of their jobs by a board of directors that declared itself anxious to resolve the staggering legal problems and position the company to concentrate on its general hospital business.

Resolving the legal problems was clearly going to be expensive. A month after the federal raids, NME agreed to pay $125 million to settle two of the insurance company lawsuits, encompassing a total of $740 million in claims. Jeffrey C. Barbakow, a former in- vestment banker and entertainment company executive who had replaced Eamer as chairman and chief executive officer, called the settlement "a major step in NME's effort to put the past behind us." One key provision of the agreement was that the insurance companies promised to "strengthen standard business relations" with NME's psychiatric hospitals.

The remaining lawsuit, involving thirteen insurance companies, was still pending as of October 1993, as was the federal criminal inquiry. In addition, about 130 individual patient suits also were pending.

In his remarks at the annual shareholders' meeting in September, Barbakow said that his "top priority" as chairman "has been on resolving the litigation relating to our psych business." Saying that "we can and must put the past behind us," the chairman described new procedures designed to "restore confidence in the company and to eliminate any concern about NME's integrity and business practices." These included assembling a "task force" to make random inspections of NME facilities; instituting independent "governing boards" at each psychiatric hospital to ensure compliance with ethical standards; tightening billing, documentation, and auditing procedures, and instituting an 800-number "hot line" for complaints or comments on patient care.

Barbakow noted that NME in 1992 had hired Richard Kusserow, a former inspector general with the U.S. Department of Health and Human Services, as its chief "compliance adviser."

NME's major corporate competitors in the psychiatric business also came in for some rough times.

In 1991, Charter Medical settled with Texas, agreeing to pay $550,000 to the state crime victims fund and to provide $1.6 million in vouchers for charity psychiatric care. The company, which operated eleven psychiatric hospitals in Texas, agreed to a number of other measures, including not using Charter counselors in public schools. Charter did not admit wrongdoing in the settlement.

In 1991, Charter Medical settled a lawsuit by Linda Eanes, the former nursing supervisor who had charged that she was fired for refusing to falsify patient records at a Charter hospital. Before the settlement was reached, a jury had characterized the hospital's actions as beyond "all possible bounds of decency" and "intolerable in a civilized community." Late the same year, after missing more than $150 million in payments on its $1.6 billion in debt, Charter filed for corporate reorganization under Chapter 11 of the federal bankruptcy code. The company successfully emerged from bankruptcy in 1992 and proclaimed in its annual report: "We are committed to dispelling the misinformation, fear and denial that surround mental illness and addictive disease by employing ethical advertising, educational, marketing and referral development practices."

In late 1991, after Community Psychiatric Centers stunned Wall Street with its announcement that its quarterly profits had plunged 98 percent because of turmoil in the psychiatric industry, analysts confirmed that CPC's decline was partly attributable to Canada's decision to stop sending psychiatric patients to American hospitals. By the first quarter of 1993, CPC's psychiatric hospital business had deteriorated to the point where the company reported a net loss and was restructuring to concentrate more on its profitable long-term acute-care hospitals and nursing homes.

HCA also cited "negative publicity surrounding the psychiatric hospital industry" for sharp declines in its psychiatric division in 1992, when the company reemerged as a publicly traded corporation and took a $365 million charge against earnings on the sale or closing of twenty-two of its psychiatric hospitals. In October 1993, HCA agreed to be acquired by another major hospital company, Columbia Healthcare Inc., in a $5.7 billion deal that would create the largest hospital chain in the world.

In Texas, Senator Moncrief called the state settlement with NME "an excellent start in the right direction," although he added, "I guess if we all had our druthers, I'd like to see them strung up by their thumbs. But that's not the name of the game here. It's to try and correct the problem."

Was the problem corrected?

That depends on how the problem is defined. Certainly, with the sheriff at the door, private psychiatric hospitals discontinued some of the most egregious abuses such as the blatant bounty-hunting that had come to light in Texas.

Yet, as anyone who watches television and reads the papers is aware, psychiatric hospitals, psychiatric wings of general hospitals, and addiction treatment centers are still eagerly trolling for customers who have insurance.

And the profession of psychiatry, which was allowed through news media indifference to shrug off the hospital scandal and blame it almost exclusively on hospital operators, continues making bold strides into the general medical field, with its plans to become a standard component of much hospital treatment. Meanwhile, the news media avidly continue to promote the claims by psychiatrists and psychologists that we are a nation suffering from an epidemic of mental illness that requires professional treatment.

In the spring of 1992 the National Association of Private Psychiatric Hospitals hired a new executive director, Robert L. Trachtenberg. Trachtenberg, who had spent the previous thirteen years as deputy administrator of the federal Alcohol, Drug Abuse, and Mental Health Administration, announced: "On any given day, more than twenty-three million Americans, including nearly eight million children, suffer from mental illnesses," with a resulting cost to the nation of $273 billion in lost productivity, accidents, crime and "other consequences"—a sum Trachtenberg claimed was four times greater than the cost of providing the necessary treatment.

Subsequently, the widely syndicated *New York Times* columnist A. M. Rosenthal extolled a comprehensive new national initiative on addiction treatment that was being led by Joseph Califano, a former U.S. health secretary: "The goal is to get America to see addiction whole, and in all its parts, to understand that ninety-five million of us are hooked on tobacco, alcohol, pot, heroin, barbiturates or crack, at a loss to the country of $300 billion a year." Califano, the director of an organization called the Center on Addiction and Substance Abuse, himself conjured up in the *Washington Post* a "sinister combine" of AIDS, alcohol, substance abuse, and tuberculosis that "threatens every man, woman, child and fetus in America" unless more money for treatment is made available, and insurance companies are required to expand coverage in such areas as addiction treatment.

In late 1992, I happened to be in Lexington, Kentucky, where I saw a local newspaper article reporting that the state department of education had given a grant to University of Kentucky psychiatrists to develop a training program to enable teachers to identify more children with "attention deficit disorder" and refer them to "outside medical experts." Beside this story was a feature article promoting a private psychiatric hospital's "Educational Resource and Technology Fair," designed so that parents could take their children for an outing while at the same time having them evaluated for attention deficit disorder by hospital personnel.

The next year, as Clinton Administration policy planners grappled with the costs of comprehensive national health care reforms, the psychiatric industry and its supporters mounted intense lobbying to include in the incipient national health plan universal coverage for sixty days of inpatient psychiatric treatment per year—a move that would bring millions of new potential paying patients into the system. As they lobbied, the insanity epidemic seemed to be worsening. In March, Daniel Goleman, a practicing psychologist who regularly covers mental-health issues in *The New York Times*, reported the latest National Institute of Mental Health study on mental illness. It concluded that *28 percent* of the adult population now suffered from a mental disorder. Goleman quoted Dr. Frederick Goodwin, the director of the National Institute of Mental Health: "It would make sense to integrate psychiatric services into general medical practice by, for example, having certain patients screened by a mental health professional" before they receive general medical treatment.

The same month, in a letter to the *Times*, Drs. Joseph T. English and John S. McIntyre, then respectively the president and president-elect of the American Psychiatric Association, proclaimed their satisfaction with the anticipated provisions in the White House plan that would expand treatment for mental illnesses and abolish the "arbitrary and artificial separation between mental illnesses and other medical illnesses," which they called "discrimination by diagnosis."

By the end of 1993, as psychiatry's lobbyists worked furiously toward ensuring that future federal health-care policy gives mental disorders "parity" with physical illnesses in insurance coverage, Goleman had discovered still more alarming news: a new study asserting that depression was vastly undertreated and cost American businesses $43.7 billion a year—as much as heart disease. Goleman quoted the NIMH's Goodwin calling depression "far more disabling than many medical disorders, including chronic lung disease, arthritis and diabetes." Meanwhile, Trachtenberg, the head of the private psychiatric hospitals' national trade organization, complained in other news accounts about "existing prejudices that have kept us from covering mental illnesses as fully as we cover physical illnesses."

Overall, the health-care industry maintains a tremendous lobbying presence in Washington and in state capitals. According to the National Health Council, the number of health-care lobby groups with offices in Washington, D.C., grew from 117 to more than 700 during the 1980s—a decade when the industry contributed a total of $60 million to candidates for Congress. At the state level, a major commercial health insurance industry lobby, the Health Insurance Association of America, reported a budget of $25 million in 1992, when its 150 full-time employees included sixteen state lobbyists. Community work is also important. Early in 1992, the Federation of American Health Systems, which represents 1,400 general, psychiatric, and other specialty hospitals, instituted a "Grassroots Business Outreach Task Force" to send speakers out to persuade local business and civic leaders to work against health-care legislation that would impose tighter restrictions on hospital spending. "We hope to mobilize small businesses in local communities to communicate to their congressmen the best way to reform the health care system," George Atkins, chairman of the task group, told the industry publication *Modern Healthcare*.

A question that many who followed the psychiatric hospital scandals asked was, why didn't the big insurance companies who were paying the exorbitant claims blow the whistle years ago? Dr. Stuckey, the psychiatrist who angrily quit as director of the alcoholism program at Fair Oaks Hospital in New Jersey, said he had wondered the same thing. Not long after he'd quit working for the hospital, Stuckey recalled, a patient whom he had treated for cocaine addiction over a two-year period at Fair Oaks brought him a stack of bills and said, "You might find these interesting." The bills totaled $375,000—and the man admitted that he was still using cocaine.

Intrigued, Stuckey took the bills to a regional headquarters of Prudential, the insurance company that had paid them. No one there batted an eye, he said. "In fact, they made jokes about a recent bill of over $100,000 submitted by Fair Oaks for a Prudential employee," Stuckey said in a letter to U.S. Rep. Patricia Schroeder, whose House Select Committee on Children, Youth, and Families held hearings into inpatient psychiatric treatment in 1992, after the Texas scandals broke. "I was dumbfounded," Stuckey wrote. "Then one of the Prudential physicians . . . pulled me aside. He said, 'Bob, don't you know we like big bills here? Big bills mean big premiums and bonuses.' "

Coincidentally, Stuckey noted, the patient with the cocaine problem "finally got straight" after attending meetings of Narcotics Anonymous—a nonprofit "twelve-step" program modeled after Alcoholics Anonymous.

Stuckey added that he once did follow-up studies on addiction-treatment patients at Fair Oaks. He said they showed that the rate of abstinence from drugs or alcohol three months after the conclusion of treatment was the same—65 percent—where the subject was in an inpatient or an outpatient program. The major differences he found were financial—outpatient treatment cost only about five percent of inpatient care—and emotional. Stuckey said he believed those in outpatient programs benefited more from being at home, and furthermore were not subject in the future to the stigma of having been in a psychiatric hospital.

"No one was watching psychiatric and substance abuse claims," said Dr. Walter Afield, the psychiatrist who founded a Tampa, Florida, firm to conduct "utilization reviews" of claims for insurance payers as they began tightening up on coverage. "It was a health benefit that paid big bucks for services rendered, and no one ever questioned the expenditures." Afield explained to Schroeder's committee that insurance companies were baffled by psychiatry.

"Psychiatry is an art form. Psychiatry is not an exact science," he said. "It generates enormous fear on the part of everybody, and the insurance companies are petrified. . . . You can't create a broken hip. However, we can create mental illness with selective and careful advertising."

"If you look at federal contracts alone, the abuse boggles the mind," said Afield. "It's hospitals and the businessmen running these hospitals that are milking the system. Usually, the psychiatrist is encouraged to go along with this revenue-generating scheme, and it's wrong. Mental-health care is determined by who is paying the bills, not by treatment needed for improvement. If you've got lots of good insurance, you're going to wind up in the hospital."

Perhaps that is inevitable in the American mental-health system, which outside of state hospitals is driven by capitalistic and not social impulses. Implicitly, such a system favors increasing supply rather than reducing demand.

To that end, new programs are still being devised to channel people with insurance into psychiatric treatment—sometimes in conjunction with general medical care. In 1992, while apparently still languishing on some mailing lists from my own short visit to Fair Oaks, I received a brochure from Morristown Memorial Hospital in New Jersey that asked, "Problems Sleeping?" If so, the hospital had a possible cure at its "Sleep Disorder Center," which featured medical evaluation during an initial overnight stay "designed to offer maximum patient comfort, centered around a living room, kitchen and cheerfully decorated bedrooms with baths." The brochure noted that most insurance plans cover the "initial consultation" and pointed out helpfully, "the Center helps patients investigate coverage amounts for further testing."

The industry refers to such programs generally as "service niches," and envisions a new era in which psychiatrists will be fully integrated into general medical care, working side-by-side with cardiologists, surgeons, gerontologists, pediatricians, and other medical specialists, in both inpatient and outpatient settings. In

December of 1992, the journal *Psychiatric Annals* declared that over half of all gastrointestinal disorders are primarily psychological in origin and "a biopsychosocially oriented psychiatrist is uniquely suited to make a positive contribution to the care of these patients."

At the same time, the counseling field long neglected by bio-psychiatrists in their rush to embrace medical science also anticipated new opportunities. Writing in *Psychiatric Quarterly*, Dr. Dennis Staton, the director of residency training at the University of North Dakota School of Medicine, predicted that in the future, "biologically oriented psychiatrists" will also work "in effective collaboration with non-physician mental health professionals," including psychologists and counselors on "multidisciplinary treatment teams" that would meet new criteria for anticipated expanded federal insurance coverage.

Problems that deeply worry most Americans, such as urban violence, have also been identified as major growth areas for biopsychiatry.

Federal policy proposals for involving psychiatrists, psychologists, and school counselors in identifying potentially violent children in the schools have been around since the Nixon administration. But the most recent one is also the most ambitious. It is called the "Youth Violence Initiative," a four-year, $400 million federal project designed to identify inner-city school children who have biological and genetic defects presumed to indicate a propensity for violence later in life.

In 1992, the National Institute of Mental Health's Dr. Goodwin explained the philosophy behind this extraordinary effort to define violent behavior as a disease-based epidemic, like smallpox or cholera, with treatment predicated on intervening among those most likely to be "infected." In a speech to the National Health Advisory Council in which he called the violence initiative the agency's "top priority," Goodwin compared the behavior of violence-prone urban children to that of jungle primates: "If you look, for example, at male monkeys, especially in the wild, roughly half of these survive to adulthood. The other half die by violence. That is the natural way of it for males, to knock each other off. . . ." Similar conditions in crime-ridden urban neighborhoods, Goodwin said, have "removed some of the civilizing evolutionary things that we have built up."

The racial overtones inherent in such a position caused a public outcry, which Goodwin downplayed while maintaining his support for the initiative. Later that year, he told the annual convention of the American Psychiatric Association that violence in America "meets the criteria of a public health epidemic." He added, "There is a genetic contribution to any social personality disorder. The environment does not cause one to be violent or to develop a criminal record if there isn't a vulnerability already there." As in any epidemic, he explained, the key response is "early detection." Goodwin suggested that elementary school teachers and counselors in "high-impact urban areas" could begin identifying violence-prone children. This might isolate 12 to 15 percent of the children, who would be placed in a program of "structured interviews" with their families. Some might eventually be enrolled in special federal day camps or be subject to psychiatric treatment, he said.

As they try to stabilize their business in the U.S. meanwhile, American psychiatric hospital companies have been expanding abroad, opening facilities in Great Britain, Spain, Japan, Canada, and other countries. In January 1993 the American Psychiatric Association's Dr. English led a delegation of prominent psychiatrists to visit Pope John Paul II in Rome, to lay groundwork for what English said he expected would be more "fruitful collaboration" between psychiatrists and the worldwide Catholic clergy, as psychiatry attempts to increase its professional activities in pastoral counseling.

But perhaps the greatest growth area seen by biopsychiatrists and their colleagues in psychology is depression.

Annually, the industry sponsors an event called National Depression Screening Day, developed jointly by the psychiatry department at Harvard Medical School and the American Psychiatric Association. In October of 1992, psychiatrists and other mental-health professionals held free screenings for depression at more than three hundred hospitals, mental-health clinics, and college health centers throughout the country. At these evaluations, people filled out a "Depression Screening Inventory," answering yes or no to twenty statements, among which were: "Morning is when I feel best" . . . "I feel hopeful about the future" . . . "My life is pretty full."

The next year the American Psychiatric Association published new guidelines to help health insurance providers to define non-recurring depression, which it characterized as feelings of "sadness, helplessness, hopelessness and irritability." According to those guidelines, 26 percent of American women and 12 percent of American men will suffer from it in their lifetime.

The horizons for biopsychiatry are broad and beckoning. In 1990 a study, hailed as a "landmark" in modern psychiatry, was published by two psychiatrists, Dr. James I. Hudson and Dr. Harrison G. Pope, Jr., in the *American Journal of Psychiatry*, the official journal of the American Psychiatric Association. In it, Hudson and Pope made the startling claim that they had identified a new, worldwide mental illness that could "emerge as one of the most widespread diseases of mankind." The authors called this global plague "affective-spectrum disorder." In their research, which was supported in part by a grant from the National Institute of Mental Health, Hudson and Pope lumped together a range of individual disorders—including major depression, obsessive-compulsive disorder, attention deficit disorder with hyperactivity and irritable bowel syndrome—in the new giant single category of affective-spectrum disorder. The implications they described were stunning. It was nothing less than a newly defined mental illness that "would represent one of the most prevalent diseases in the population." Furthermore, given the nature of this disorder, spouses, children and other close relatives are likely to be afflicted. As a result, Pope declared in a 1992 interview, affective-spectrum disorder "may affect a third of the population of the world."

Those are pretty heady claims to challenge, for a reporter who only came to learn anything about this subject because he felt ripped off by a hospital where he had gone for information.

I claim no expertise whatever in medicine—psychiatric or otherwise. Nor do I automatically accept the righteousness of antipsychiatry and antimedication crusaders, some of whom seem to be partly driven by their own modern brand of Puritan morality. I have walked down too many New York City streets, witnessing the wretchedness of the deranged, to believe glib assertions that there is no such thing as mental illness. Their misery is a constant reminder that as we divert large sums into psychiatric treatment for the "worried well"—as psychiatrists rush to treat "diseases that do not exist," in the words of Dr. Szasz, psychiatry's chief iconoclast—we have abandoned many of the chronically and severely mentally ill, the ones who tend to be poor and difficult to manage, the ones who need help most.

Still, it is apparent to me that many Americans—children among them—are functioning better today because of quality psychiatry and addiction treatment. And while Prozac sounds to me a lot like controlled drug addiction for the affluent, a kind of cocaine without the risks, who am I to denounce the claims that "cosmetic psychopharmacology" can bring a fuller and even more vibrant life to some? That is certainly for them to decide.

Furthermore, I have nothing but admiration for the millions of people who have managed to overcome drinking and drug problems through nonprofit programs such as Alcoholics Anonymous. May they live and prosper, whatever their "higher force" may be. And may all of us "self-curers" prosper along with them.

When I began this book, I knew that it had to be essentially about money. So let me now add my last two cents to the debate over health care that will occupy us in this country for the rest of the twentieth century. It is merely common street advice on how to avoid being hustled: Keep an eye on who approaches you, and a hand on your wallet.

INDEX

INDEX